OVERWHELMED

OVERWHELMED

One Woman's Journey with Breast Cancer

KAREN L. NORTON

TATE PUBLISHING & Enterprises

Published by Tate Publishing & Enterprises, LLC
127 E. Trade Center Terrace | Mustang, Oklahoma 73064 USA
1.888.361.9473 | www.tatepublishing.com

Tate Publishing is committed to excellence in the publishing industry. The company reflects the philosophy established by the founders, based on Psalm 68:11,
"The Lord gave the word and great was the company of those who published it."

Book design copyright © 2010 by Tate Publishing, LLC. All rights reserved.
Cover design by Kellie Southerland
Interior design by Joey Garrett

Published in the United States of America

ISBN: 978-1-61739-068-5
1. Religion / Christian Life / Women's Issues
2. Health & Fitness / Diseases / Cancer
10.11.16

DEDICATION

This book is dedicated to my loving husband, Ken, and our two daughters, Allison and Mackenzie, who constantly gave me a reason for surviving breast cancer.

PROLOGUE

I couldn't believe it. I was in shock. I hurried out of the hospital clinic, walking as quickly as I could to my car. Where could I go? Where could I run? Who could I lean on at a time like this?

To go home immediately was out of the question. My husband, Ken, had been enduring unemployment for eighteen months. No matter how many résumés he sent out or odd jobs he found, nothing was steady or permanent. We were living on my part-time salary as a music pastor. We had gone through all of our savings and wondered how much longer we would be able to keep our house. We knew we were in God's will, but now this?

Ken was beyond stressed out. He had been promised a job with a start-up company, with which we could live anywhere. We lived from one week to the next, in anticipation that this was the week for his job to materialize. Month after month went by. Both of us were about at our limits of what we could handle. We were going deeper in debt, even in the midst of our new life that we had come to love since moving in January 1999 from Quincy, Illinois.

As I began to drive out of the hospital clinic parking lot, tears soaked my face. I began to shake all over, even though it wasn't cold on this spring day in the year 2000. The grass was finally green, the flowers were beginning to pop out, but I was not aware of the beauty around me. I knew in my heart that this would happen to me sooner or later, but now, why now of all times? I had a good chance of this occurring since my mother's younger sister had fought it several years earlier. Statistics reveal the likelihood through the mother's genes. This was *not* a good time. I did not have any control over *when*. It seemed I was losing control of my life. Had God forgotten about us? Had He forsaken us? Were we being punished for some unknown reason? How much more distress would God allow us to go through?

So many questions raced through my mind. What was going to happen? What would we do? How could I handle this? Would this affect my position at the church as music pastor? Would the senior pastor I was serving with understand? Would the congregation understand?

Our two little precious daughters, Allison, almost three, and Mackenzie, twenty months, were too young to understand what was happening. How could their mother go through something like this? It seemed they needed my undivided attention twenty-four hours a day. Ken was home, constantly on the Internet seeking employment possibilities. I could not bother him with this. I was determined to be strong yet I felt so helpless.

I had just been told by the radiologist I had the beginning stages of breast cancer. He asked how that made me feel. I told him I was thankful it was caught early. I knew that early detection was one of the best keys to survival. Deep down, I knew I was just trying to cover up my true feelings with someone I did not even know. Come on, what was I supposed to say? Did he expect me to become hysterical?

I was forty-one years old. I had been so busy over the last several years. I had married Ken at the age of thirty-five. We waited two and a half years before having Allison Grace. Mackenzie Joy came fourteen and a half months later. Our family was complete; God gave us two girls—just what we wanted! Their middle names spoke of what we believed we would always have in our home—grace and joy. More than ever, we needed *grace* and *joy* now.

We moved two hundred miles to take a music pastor position when Mackenzie was a little over three months old. We had so much sickness the first few months after we moved; it seemed that our whole family would never again be well all at the same time. Flu viruses occurred endlessly, traveling to each person in our family. Our bodies needed to adjust to living in a different environment.

Later, Mackenzie gave us a scare when she was nine months old. Thoughts came to our minds at that time that we were going to lose her. We watched her little body become frail and her eyes become sunken. She had become dehydrated from days of diarrhea, landing her in the hospital for twenty-four hours to replenish her little body of fluids. Mackenzie became healthy once again and full of vitality.

Now it was almost a year later. I had breast cancer. Cancer. The big C. The word that puts fear into one's heart and mind. The word that makes you think of your own mortality. The word that changes the way you look at the rest of your life. The word that happens to *other people, not to me.* After all, I grew up with the anthem, "I am woman, hear me roar... If I have to, I can do anything. I am strong, I am invincible, I am woman."

The ten-minute drive across town was a blur as I faced the news of breast cancer. I began retracing the events as they led up to this new day. I had gone to my family doctor, as I was having problems with hemorrhoids. She gave me a complete physical. I agreed to have a mammogram, for I had not had one since my baseline mammogram at the age of thirty-five. The baseline mammogram is the first mammogram a woman has. It is recommended by the American Cancer Society for women between the ages of thirty-five and forty. My baseline had shown some questionable calcifications then. Now as my doctor called me a few days later after the mammogram, requesting my presence back for more pictures, I did not have a good feeling. She was hopeful, saying it was a routine thing to do. I was large busted and mammograms sometimes have difficulty finding everything in large-busted women. Facts were facts; I was large-busted. I had always been large busted and having children only increased this endowment. I joked about my large breasts, often making comments about eagerly awaiting heaven where no bras would be worn at all! How I had longed for that freedom!

Here I was with breast cancer. This was no laughing matter now! The abnormal calcifications were shown in the left breast. The radiologist had told me I would have a biopsy to expunge the cancer.

What was I going to do? I was thankful we had taken out health insurance for our family from my part-time income. I believed my strong faith in God would pull me through anything. Little did I know what lay ahead in the months to come. How my faith was tested, yet strengthened, would prove God's loving kindness and faithfulness to me. Yes, I believed God could heal me so I would not have to go through breast cancer. God can do anything, and I really believed that. Somehow, some way, I believed there was a divine purpose in going through breast cancer.

CHAPTER ONE

Fear and trembling overwhelm me, and I can't
stop shaking.

Psalm 55:5

I found myself in the driveway of my new
friend, Linda. She lived close by and on my way home.
Still shaking, I got out of the car and stumbled to the
door to ring the doorbell. As I waited for Linda to
answer the door, I was nearly frantic. *She's just got to be
home,* I thought as I rang the doorbell again and again.
No answer. Determined, I tried various means of making my presence known. I finally came enough to my
senses to realize she couldn't hear my banging or the
doorbell, so I ran around to the back of the house and
scratched on the screen window. This got Linda's attention as I saw her peek through the window, motioning
me back to the front door.

Linda took one look at me and asked, "What's
going on?" I blurted out that I had just come from hav-

ing my second mammogram. The radiologist told me I had the beginning stages of breast cancer.

Linda invited me in to talk about what all this meant and what was the next step. Through tears, I poured out my emotions. Then strength began to resurface in me. I knew, with God's help, I could face whatever I had to go through in the next few weeks and months. I was thankful to have a friend with whom I could vent my emotions before facing my family in our already stress-filled home.

Head up and shoulders back, I left Linda's house to go home and share this news with my husband. I dreaded telling him, but I knew I had to be open and share this with him. I didn't know how he would take this news. He was already burdened with trying to find employment. This would definitely add to the stress level for him.

We had always shared everything in our marriage. We believed trust in a marriage is built on open communication. Get the feelings out in the open and then we will deal with it. Sure, we had our disagreements from time to time, like any married couple, but we always sought to resolve our issues through openness and honesty.

I braced myself as I entered our home. Upon seeing their mommy and getting their hugs, Allie and Mackenzie ran off to play. With two little girls born closely together, they were instant playmates. Ken and I sat on the love seat in the living room. As I began to share with him the outcome of the second mammogram and what it meant, Ken lovingly took hold of my hand. He was not surprised. I think the Lord had prepared him for this moment. That was a relief to me. He reassured me we would get through this difficult time together with God's help and strength. We always believed that nothing ever happened to us but that God could use it for His ultimate glory if we allowed ourselves to be His vessels. We agreed we did not want to wait around, but to go ahead and meet with the surgeon and schedule the biopsy as quickly as possible.

The next few days seemed like a bad dream, as I proceeded with what must be done. There were people I had to tell, the first one being my mother. This was a most unpleasant task, as my mother had survived uterine cancer in 1993. We thought we were going to lose her at that time, when her kidneys started to fail. Miraculously, the Lord brought her through this. She had been on kidney dialysis, but to this day has had no more problems with her kidneys and is in good health. My mother had a brother die of cancer in 1979. Her sister had survived breast cancer in 1978.

I also had to share with my own siblings, two brothers and a sister, what was going on in my life. We are a close family, so something this significant in my life could not be swept under the rug. It hit my older sister, Pat, as she and I are close in spite of the ten years' difference in our ages. When cancer hits a sibling, it makes one realize it could hit as well. My two brothers, Bill and Dan, tend to be stoic, so it was hard to tell how the news affected them. Bill, my older brother, is married to Jane. Jane had lost both of her parents to cancer when she was a teenager. She knew cancer firsthand and knew not to mess around with it. Since Dan had never married, he lived with our parents. Our mother gave Dan the news of my breast cancer. His comments regarding this news showed some concern for my well-being.

There was the church to consider. Being on staff, I first told the senior pastor and his wife, Ed and Judy Aubuchon. They are a couple who believe strongly in prayer. I knew I would have tremendous prayer support through them. I had known and worked with them off and on throughout my years of ministry. We had a strong friendship. Upon telling them the news, they were most gracious and compassionate. We joined together in prayer, believing God to have His perfect will in this situation.

I chose to tell the choir separately and first before the congregation. The choir supported me in several ways. They were always such a tremendous blessing to me. I told them I did not want any sympathy but that we would continue serving the Lord to the best of our ability. They respected my wishes and lovingly kept on singing and ministering to the Lord, Sunday after Sunday.

How do you tell a congregation you have breast cancer? As a minister, I knew I lived my life in a fishbowl. The congregation had to know what was happening to me in order to know the best possible way to pray for my family and myself. They were already praying for Ken to find work. I hated to burden them with anything else. As I shared with the congregation, I found added strength through the prayer they gave my family and me continuously. If I had to have cancer, this was the time to have it. In this loving congregation, I had a good support system. They volunteered right and left to help our family in the midst of our crisis.

I was so stubborn and self-sufficient that I did not want any help around the house. I just wanted to get the cancer out of my body and get on with my life. I was not happy about the timing of this ordeal. We were making progress in the church, tearing down strongholds, when the news of the cancer came. It was just like the enemy of our souls to set up roadblocks in our moving forward for the Lord. This did make the congregation, along with the choir, determined to press on and through the enemy's tactics. The devil may attempt to do evil in our bodies, but God is always victorious through the shed blood of Jesus!

I did not like anything slowing me down. I did not want to sit around feeling sorry for myself or letting others feel sorry for me. I was not going to die. I was determined to live. Being an ordained minister with the Assemblies of God since 1987, I had a calling on my life that would not let me be idle nor dissuaded from my life's work. Most importantly, God had brought into my life a husband and two little girls that made me determined to beat this cancer, whatever sacrifice it took on my part.

I had a passion for serving the Lord, and I was blessed with a husband that complemented my ministry. I had everything going for me and then breast cancer happened. On one hand, I had resentment toward it and God. On the other hand, I trusted the Lord with my life and knew He could use me to help others going through the same thing. I struggled with mixed emotions, and there were plenty of them!

At times like this, people will give all kinds of advice on what to do or not do. I believe in always listening to people and their counsel, but ultimately it is best to hear personally from God. It was during these initial days of breast cancer that God revealed to me a vision of my path of life and what I must endure for His sake. This helped me in the weeks and months ahead.

CHAPTER TWO

When I am overwhelmed, you alone know the way I should turn. Wherever I go, my enemies have set traps for me.

Psalm 142:3

This path of life was in full Technicolor, God's way. I saw a brown, dirt path that started at the bottom, right where I was, with a slight curve as it meandered up a hill. One could not see over the hill, however. There were trees on the sides of the path and greenery everywhere. The greenery was beautiful. It reminded me of the green grass of Ireland when Ken took me there on a business trip in the fall of 1997. Allison was just two and a half months old when we traveled there for a week. I was enamored by the green grass in Ireland, much like I was admiring the greenery now along this path God had placed before me in my vision.

In my stubbornness, I told God I did not want to go on this path, as I did not know where it would take me. He instructed me that one step at a time I would climb this hill, even though I could not see over the hill. I told Him I was not comfortable with this. I wanted to see the full scope of this path before taking it. I thought that was only fair since He was asking this of me. He gently spoke to me, "Trust Me. Trusting is when you do not see or know what lies ahead, but you proceed out of obedience and reverence for Me."

Next, I argued with the Lord that I wanted to turn around and go back. I wanted to pretend this breast cancer did not exist. I was scared. I did not like what was happening in my life. I had no control in the matter. I did not have time for this. It was an interruption in my life for which I had not bargained. I thought a better time for this to happen, if it had to happen, would be after the girls were grown. We always think we know what is best for us. That is when we take the Lord out of the equation of our lives. The Lord again spoke lovingly to me that I could not turn around and go back, as the brown path disappeared behind me as I walked the path. I could not believe this! *There was no turning back.* Those words stung. I had to face reality. Pretending it did not exist was not an option. I wanted options! Cancer had been found. Confronting adversity in life is never a pleasant task but is necessary for growth. I must walk the path and carry on. I could not even stand still. I would get weary by doing so.

Still trying the Lord's patience, I asked if I could step off of the brown path and on to the greenery. It looked so tempting and beautiful. Why take an ugly dirt path when I could be walking in the greenery? What harm was there in this? Could this be an option? The Lord once again spoke to my heart in this vision and simply said no without an explanation. It was the parental kind of no that He gave me. I knew not to push for any explanation. I knew the story of Adam and Eve and did not want to be disobedient (see Genesis 3).

How ironic that the brown, dirt path represented my life. The Bible says we are but dust. From the ground, we were created (Genesis 2:7). So much of our lives is dirt and filth; we are nothing in comparison to our Lord Jesus Christ, who is perfect in every way!

The Lord went on to tell me that my physical healing would come as I went through these various elements of breast cancer: the biopsy, the lumpectomy, the radiation, and taking the prescription of Tamoxifen. The radiation treatments and the Tamoxifen were preventative measures of combating breast cancer. There are never any guarantees, but the fact that the breast cancer had been found in its early stages was hopeful. It was important to me that cancer never again entered my life. However, I knew I was young and the odds were against me for having a recurrence of the cancer.

I finally came to the realization that there was no choice in the matter. God had clearly spelled everything out to me in this vision of the path. This was the path of life that God had ordained for me. I knew this was my cup, my cross, and I must accept it. Accepting it was one thing; liking it was another. Neither could be accomplished overnight. It would take much time.

Everyone must find his or her own path of life. It is not the same for everyone. We are all so very different. What is good for one may not be good for another. Through seeking God and His will, one will find his path of life. The Scripture that God gave me in reference to this path of life was Psalm 16:11: "You have made known to me the path of life; you will fill me with joy in your presence, with eternal pleasures at your right hand" (NIV).

It wasn't until a year and a half later when our family was vacationing in Missouri that God turned my vision into reality. As a family, we were hiking in the woods when suddenly we came upon the very vision that God had given me. I was ecstatic and asked Ken to photograph this path for me. It meant so much to me, as I knew there was significance beyond my understanding. It was at this time that God revealed to me that the tempting greenery along the sides of the path was *poison ivy!* The poison ivy represented sin and disobedience. The Lord had been teaching me about obedience since the beginning of the breast cancer.

Through the next several days, I had the biopsy taken, which did indeed reveal cancer. It was then determined that a lumpectomy be performed, as there was more cancer. It was a different kind of cancer, however. I did not know how much cancer would be found. As a precaution, the surgeon deemed it best to remove all of the lymph nodes along with the breast tissue.

As the anesthesia began to take effect for the lumpectomy, music flooded my being. Music has played in my heart and mind throughout the course of my life. This day was no exception. I began to softly hum and then sing the chorus: "Jesus, lover of my soul. Jesus, I will never let you go. You've taken me from the miry clay. You've set my feet upon the rock, and now I know. I love you; I need you. Though my world may fall, I'll never let you go. My Savior, my closest friend. I will worship You until the very end."

I drifted away to awaken a few hours later with pain from the incisions. I was told the cancer had been totally expunged. There was no cancer found in the lymph nodes. I was very thankful for this.

Quite often, I see humor in life's experiences. This was one of those times. My two three- and four-inch incisions had staples binding them. This reminded me of railroad tracks bypassing each other. I found myself fascinated by this. Even though the staples were painful, I could laugh at the *forever* scars this would create on my body. Since Ken was a photographer, it seemed fitting that he should photograph my incisions. After all, I would never be physically the same again. He complied and took photos—memories of God's faithfulness to our lives!

My breast cancer was determined to be stage one. My chance of survival was nearly one hundred percent. I downplayed the seriousness of this disease. I can be flippant in times of crises. I told myself this was only a taste in comparison to what so many men and women face when confronting the reality of cancer. Perhaps I was still in a state of denial.

Cancer is such an ugly word. Unless diagnosed, we are not even aware of its existence. Hidden deep on the inside, we cannot see the destruction being wreaked on our bodies.

Even though the prognosis was good, radiation was still recommended just to be on the safe side. There could be stray cancer cells lurking in my breast tissue that the radiation would surely destroy. For now, I had to take the time to heal before starting radiation therapy.

CHAPTER THREE

From the ends of the earth, I cry to you for help when my heart is overwhelmed. Lead me to the towering rock of safety.

Psalm 61:2

I **was so** thankful I had married a self-sufficient man who could cook and take care of changing diapers. I did not enjoy cooking or being domestic. My focus was on being a minister to a congregation. I was driven to watching people become all they could be for Christ's sake and His kingdom.

Ken was constantly on the Internet or making phone calls, looking for possible full-time employment or even temporary employment. With one eye on the computer and the other eye on our two little daughters, he was a busy man. The stress level was tremendous. He was concerned about my well-being, yet feeling helpless in providing a living for his family. It was times like these when we were tempted to question the hand of God. And we did.

On a scale of one to ten, with ten being the greatest level of stress, we each scored a ten. We were stressed out with our concerns. One day Ken and I found ourselves disagreeing over something trivial. We realized then that we were unable to comfort and encourage each other as we both had our own burdens to carry. And how heavy those burdens were to bear.

Allie was barely potty-trained, and Mackenzie was months from tackling that feat. Toys were scattered across the house. We had a bay window in our living room adjacent to the sofa where I would lie. The girls would use the bay window as a stage to perform shows for me. In spite of the heartaches we were dealing with, we strove to maintain stability in our girls' lives as well as our own. Amidst the turmoil, the girls continued to be a source of joy and laughter, constant in-house entertainment, as it were. My incisions were referred to as "Mommy's owies" to help explain to the girls the seriousness of the matter. Though their youthful curiosity was boundless, I was constantly amazed at their capacity for concern and compassion.

We also experienced God's grace with the church family. I continued with my responsibilities at the church, leading the praise and worship for the Sunday services and directing the choir. I continued with all the musical preparation that goes into leading people. I knew in my heart what God expected of me. It had nothing to do with giving up responsibility. It was all about accepting what I had to endure and being an example to the congregation.

Though hired as part-time, my schedule was full at the church. From the first mammogram on April

27 to the diagnosis and ensuing lumpectomy on May 16, I was barely out of the hospital when the church's annual mother-daughter banquet was held on May 19. Determination and the grace of God made it a matter of importance to attend the banquet. I knew that God did not want me to let up with any of my church obligations, so I was there at the mother-daughter banquet with my mother and two daughters. It was a testimony of God's kindness and love.

The outward scars from the lumpectomy and lymph nodes were healing nicely. Inwardly, I was churning. I was a mess. So much was on my mind. Ken's need to find full-time employment to support our family was uppermost in my mind. Then there was the question, was I really cancer free? Or would cancer again rear its ugly head sometime in the future? On top of these concerns, our financial situation had gone from bad to worse. We had gone through all of our savings, even our 401(k). Our two credit cards were at their limits, and we were about to lose our house because we could not make the mortgage payments. Oh, how we loved this house! God knew what we needed when He directed us to this house! We were forced to write a letter of hardship to the bank that held our mortgage loan in order to keep our house. It was all a very humbling experience. The Lord does not like pride in any of us. He will allow us to go through circumstances to prune the pride that can sprout like weeds in our lives. This was our time of painful but necessary pruning.

Ken and I trusted God and relied on Him. Well, that was always our intent and desire, but through this time, we learned how reliant on our Lord we truly were. We asked ourselves the question: Would we have moved the two hundred miles here if we had known all that was going to happen to our family? We could honestly answer yes to this difficult question. Our lives were miserable before moving, as we were sensing God's direction elsewhere. When a person finds God's will, it does not matter what obstacles are encountered. God's grace is sufficient through the storms of life. Just as a storm comes along, it also passes in a matter of time. It is what you do during the storm that counts. Does the storm bring turmoil or does the storm bring peace? Does the storm bring darkness or does the storm bring impossible light? Does the storm show how vulnerable we really are or does the storm show where our security lies? It is ultimately our responsibility to learn the life's lessons that come as a result of the storms.

As time drew closer to the beginning of radiation treatments, I had to keep my focus on the vision that the Lord had given to me. I did not want to experience the radiation treatments. I had had the lumpectomy and the cancer was removed. Why couldn't I get on with my life? Why was it such a big deal to have the radiation treatments? Out of obedience, I knew I had to surrender my life and my will to the Lord on a daily basis. I needed to complete the requirements He had asked of me.

I have been a Christian for what seems to be my entire life. I had grown up in church and even had seventeen years of perfect attendance in Sunday school in my childhood years. Apparently, it did not matter how good, religious, spiritual or godly I was; breast cancer had still invaded my body.

It was at this time the Lord directed my attention to a passage in the Bible that has become quite popular over the last several years. These verses gave me focus, strength for the journey, and comfort in the midst of this ordeal. Jeremiah 29:11–13 became the scripture I quoted to myself every day and eventually memorized: "For I know the plans I have for you, says the Lord. They are plans for good and not for disaster, to give you a future and a hope. In those days when you pray, I will listen. If you look for me wholeheartedly, you will find me."

I needed to hide this scripture in my heart, knowing that God would see me through this trial. I had often told myself that God has a plan. That does not mean a partial plan, but a complete plan. His plan exists for my good. Years before, when Ken called me on the telephone and told me that he had bad news, the Lord spoke to my heart and said, "I have a plan." This bad news was that he had been laid off by his employer. This was not the kind of news one likes to hear with daughters who are sixteen months old and six weeks old. Baby formula and diapers are daily expenses with babies this close together in age.

This news came on Ken's fifth anniversary of being with the company. Ironically, Ken still received his five-year gift signifying the company's appreciation of his years of dedicated service. We could have adopted the bitter attitude of "That's a *fine* way of showing your appreciation!" Instead, the Lord spoke softly to our hearts that He had a plan. It was because of Ken's losing his job that we had moved here. God worked through this to move us to a new location and ministry. We knew once again that God had a plan in this breast cancer.

CHAPTER FOUR

Please listen and answer me, for I am overwhelmed by my troubles.

Psalm 55:2

On Thursday morning, June 1, 2000, I
had my first meeting with the radiologist. I was truly
blessed with another fine physician. He had a level of
calmness and peace that were instrumental in making
me feel at ease.

I have always endeavored to maintain a calm facade
that usually serves to mask my naturally high-strung
nature. However, I felt that facade crumble as the doctor drew pictures on a paper for me, and the enormity
of this breast cancer and impending radiation therapy
came crashing down on me.

Radiation is a science and had to be carried out as
such. I again met with the radiologist on Tuesday, June
13, to get my "dots" put on my left breast. This was a
guideline for the radiation to be administered into my
body. Precision was of utmost importance.

Finally, the first day of radiation treatments arrived on Monday, June 26. My support system was strong: I had Allie and Mackenzie with me to focus on, and my dear friend Linda accompanied me. I did not want to burden Ken with this added stress, as he was so desperately seeking employment. I had learned years before a woman should look to a girlfriend for emotional support and not always put that responsibility upon her husband.

When my name was called, I left my support system behind in the waiting room, and I was ushered by a young woman who was to become my angel in disguise. As I finished changing into my hospital gown, tears welled up inside me. I was not left alone for long in my tearful stage. I was feeling so rebellious about starting these radiation treatments. If I could have kicked and screamed my way out of doing this, I would have. I was not looking forward to the summer months. For all practical purposes, I knew my summer was ruined. I would be tied to these radiation treatments five days a week. I did take pleasure, however, in the fact that those dearest to me made sure the experience was as enjoyable as possible. My support system assisted me along this path of life that I had to endure for His glory.

My angel in disguise asked me how I was doing, and I told her in no uncertain terms that I did not want to be there, but I was doing this in obedience to my heavenly Father. She explained to me she could only be there by the grace of God herself, doing this job. She gave me a hug and just held me for a moment to reassure me. It was then I knew God had sent her my way as added reinforcement. The strange thing was I did not see her again until several weeks later, close to the end of my treatments. During her absence, I had imagined that she truly was an angel in disguise.

In the radiation room, two technicians set everything up before leaving the room to administer the radiation laser. I was placed on a table, with my arms positioned above my head. The technicians would mechanically raise the table to the location necessary for the radiation laser to hit locations accordingly throughout my body. As I looked directly above me to the ceiling that was an open grid system, there was an angel figurine. It was like a Christmas tree ornament and was positioned so I could focus on it. I knew God's angels were with me in this lonely room. I had to hold still and hold my breath. In a matter of seconds, the radiation laser had penetrated, completing its assignment for the day with this patient. Then the technicians reappeared, lowering the table so I could freely leave and get on with my day.

From that time on, I always felt God's presence and peace in the radiation room. Not only that, I knew He had an angel with me there in that room. On more than one occasion, out of the corner of my eye, I caught a glimpse of a much larger image of the little angelic figurine. I was most fascinated by the presence of the angel in there with me. I had often heard stories of others who had reported seeing God's angels, but I had never before encountered one myself. I am convinced, even though I cannot back it up with scriptural reference, that God allows us to see our own personal angel during traumatic times in our lives. Angels are always with us, but at special times when we most need reassuring, they are made visible to the naked eye.

After the first day of radiation, I began to regain some of my self-reliance. I started to think this wasn't going to be such a big deal after all. Radiation treatments were not painful! This was a short-lived delusion; in a matter of a few days, the daily fatigue had set in. I needed a traveling companion, so most of the time Linda would accompany me the seventy miles roundtrip to the radiation treatment center. If she could not make the trip, other arrangements were made. I was always grateful for the moral support. I wanted to drive myself, but the fatigue became such a factor that Linda would have to drive us home. Allie and Mackenzie would join us, giving their dad some alone time to pursue employment opportunities.

It got to the point where I was so fatigued all the time that it was like going without sleep for a week. In reality, that was not the case. Being fatigued like that made it difficult to function around the house or at the church. The grace of God carried me every step of the way. There would be times when different ones from the church would want to cook a meal for us or take care of our laundry. I was so determined to do it all that many people were robbed of a blessing because of my stubbornness. Ken was good about doing things like vacuuming and cooking, while I managed to do the laundry and the inevitable cleanup from Ken's cooking.

No amount of rest or sleep would keep the fatigue away. I felt like a walking zombie. I would take daily naps usually when the girls would take their naps.

Another passage of Scripture that I incorporated in my daily devotional time was Psalm 91. This had been a Scripture that had helped a friend of mine when she went through breast cancer. It truly ministered to me, and I latched on to it during those days of radiation treatment. It is a psalm that speaks particularly to us when we are in danger. My very being did indeed feel as though I were in danger. Cancer had taken up residence in my body!

It wasn't long into the days and weeks of the radiation treatments before the Lord showed me another vision of His provision regarding the significance of the radiation treatments. He showed me that the radiation table that I had to lie on was like laying my all on the altar of God. The altar is indicative of dying to self and allowing the Lord to change and cleanse us of our sins. It is then we are molded into His image. We have to come willingly to the altar for God to change us. I had to come willingly to the radiation table for the radiation to be applied. The light of the radiation represented the light of God shining in me, expelling the cancer. Not only was the physical cancer being eradicated, but the spiritual cancer as well. The light of the red laser was symbolic of the blood of Jesus, washing and cleansing me of all sin, the spiritual cancer lurking in my body. I became excited with this vision of how God was purifying me as I allowed Him to take control. It was at this time I learned to surrender my all to Him. I now wanted to go through the radiation treatments and did so willingly. My desire had always been to be more like Jesus.

The Lord never seems to be early, nor is He late. He is always just on time. He never allows us to go through more than we can handle. At times, we may question whether we can go through various situations, but He knows we can. His ways are best. On Monday, July 31, 2000, Ken began full-time employment with a local telephone company as a data network engineer. Linda and I had stood together in agreement, trusting God, that Ken would get this job. After struggling for so long, Ken had been beaten down, and he was no longer hopeful. The Lord came through for Ken and our family in the nick of time. Ken was employed with a new industry! He had several years of experience in the broadcast industry and felt most comfortable there. I had been prompting him that God wanted him in the telecommunications industry. I saw this as a progressive industry. Ken is gifted in learning quickly. The first several days of employment were a whirlwind in our household as he studied and researched, coming to know the ins and outs of the industry.

The pieces of the puzzle began to fit together. The job Ken had been promised with the start-up company when we had moved here and his preparation with that actually dovetailed with his new employment. All of the daily, weekly, and monthly frustrations of holding on for that promised job now dissolved as we saw how God had used those times for our good. Romans 8:28 says, "And we know that God causes everything to work together for the good of those who love God and are called according to his purpose for them." Still, questions flooded our minds. Why now? Why didn't this job materialize *before* the breast cancer? Or, why couldn't this job wait to start *after* I finished the radiation treatments? Questions like these should always prompt us to trust the Lord and His ways. Proverbs 3:5–6 says, "Trust in the LORD with all your heart; do not depend on your own understanding. Seek his will in all you do, and he will show you which path to take." We would never completely understand God's ways, but we could trust Him.

What He did reveal to us was that this was His timing. The company Ken started working for was another start-up company that was just getting its feet on the ground. We also could see God's hand in Ken being home with Allie and Mackenzie during their most formative years as a good thing.

At last, we could breathe a sigh of relief as Ken went off to work every day, knowing that more income was coming into our household.

CHAPTER FIVE

Don't let the floods overwhelm me, or the deep waters swallow me, or the pit of death devour me.

Psalm 69:15

We soon learned our problems were not completely over, however. Digging our way out of the debt we had incurred was going to take some time. It seemed like a case of two steps forward, one step back, as we inched our way into a normal way of living again with Ken employed. I was used to having Ken around the house to help out with the girls, the cooking, and the vacuuming. Now I was on my own. When Ken came home from work in the evening, I knew he was tired. He would help out with the evening meal preparations, but there were times we would fuss at each other due to our own tiredness and what we were individually dealing with. He was tired from learning a new line of work and the pressure involved with that, along with being the main income provider once again. I was tired from the radiation treatments, taking care of two toddlers, managing a home, plus my music pastor position at the church. The medical bills seemed endless with four physicians involved, radiation treatments, medications, and hospital expenses. It would take years to recover from this setback of Ken not being employed for twenty-one months. We began making minimal monthly payments on all the medical bills.

The radiation treatments had affected my body in so many ways. The fatigue caused by the radiation was only the beginning. Because of my fair complexion, the radiation treatments soon turned into a bad sunburn on the bottom of my left breast. It was a continual burning, day after day. It was not a typical sunburn, in that it would heal and become normal again. It was constant and increasingly painful. It was not a normal location for a sunburn. I had never before exposed that part of my body to the sun. Once the area was burned, then it began to itch. This caused a great deal of discomfort. I notified the radiologist at one of my routine visits with him. As a result, the density of the radiation treatments had to be diminished. By this point in time, this was acceptable as the radiation was getting into the body as necessary.

My skin was so irritated that I began to go braless. Now, for a large-busted woman, this was not an easy task. Trying to hide the fact that I was going braless, I wore jackets over my blouses or dresses. My breasts were so large they hung to my waist. I just wanted to be comfortable as I was recovering. This seemed to be impossible. However, I was to the point I did not care what people thought, as I was engrossed in the process of surviving and conquering breast cancer. This was my main focus. On the other hand, it was enjoyable not to be harnessed with a bra. I had to see the humor in this life's circumstance.

Another aspect of the humor I discovered in this was how the lumpectomy had reshaped my left breast. Thankfully, it was not noticeable to the human eye. My right breast hung down, but my left breast was actually somewhat perky. The two breasts looked like misaligned automobile headlights.

Because I was constantly extremely tired, I would say things that were hilarious to others and to me. Words and sentences do not always come together in the order intended. For instance, I would say something like this: "He blew her bluff," or, "I swallowed it hook, bait, and sinker," or, "If the truth fits, wear it!" or, "It was another link in my fence." It was not uncommon for me to mix metaphors while I was dopey from the radiation treatments. To those closest to me, I was often a source of amusement.

I was thankful to the Lord that He helped me with my attitude throughout the radiation treatments. It was vital that my attitude continue to be positive in the healing process. I knew this would prove to be tremendously cathartic. I had watched various people in the ministry as well as my own family endured the experience of cancer; some had a will and desire to live as well as a good attitude while others just wanted to die.

Finally, my last day of radiation treatments came on August 10, 2000. The six and a half weeks of radiation had been a grueling process. It seemed that the treatments would never be finished. Day after day, the treatments went on and on. It was like riding a carousel endlessly. I barely knew what I was doing as the fatigue had set in long before.

The relationships I had developed with the radiation technicians had to end now. The radiation treatment center was such a caring place with compassionate employees. It truly was a pleasant experience during an unpleasant time in my life. I would have my six-month checkups and mammograms here at the center from now on and then I would see the personnel. Going to the radiation treatments had become an emotional attachment that I had to leave behind so that I could get on with my life. I was not prepared for the abruptness that this entailed. It seemed like the umbilical cord was being cut without my permission. These technicians had been my support system, my cheerleaders on a daily basis. Suddenly, that portion of the breast cancer experience was over.

I thought it would be simple to get on with my life. It wasn't the emotional attachments that were a problem, however. It was the physical aspect and the aftereffects of the radiation on my body. I had to regain my strength. The fatigue took awhile to work its way out of me.

I became increasingly aware of the shortness of breath I was encountering. I had pain in my left breast and arm that felt like I was having the lumpectomy performed all over again. I learned later this was normal, as nerve endings have to either die off or live. As a result, this can mimic the pain of the actual surgery.

I started having problems with my eyes. The thought crossed my mind that I needed a new prescription for my contacts. I went to my optometrist and discovered through a process lasting several weeks that my old contacts had damaged my eyes. This might not have happened if I had been able to keep my yearly appointment that was scheduled at the time the breast cancer was detected. I had to deal with my attitude once again, as I felt bitterness toward the cancer rise like bile inside of me. My eyes had to take some time to heal before getting new contacts, which meant I had to wear my glasses all the time. All I could think about was what else I was going to have to endure.

As far as medications, in June 2000 I had been put on Tamoxifen to help ward off any cancer cells entering the breast tissue again. Being on the Tamoxifen, I started feeling slight hot flashes. I was most intrigued with this phenomenon. I had always been around other women who experienced hot flashes and knew how much women seemed to hate them. I, on the other hand, did not hate them, as they were not bad at all. I did not have a sense of feeling normal again, but believed that the worst was behind me and that surely I was on the road to recovery.

Autumn was ushered in during this time of recovery after the radiation treatments. The ongoing shortness of breath and lack of energy seemed to linger. This was not pleasing to me, as I wanted my life back. Mentally, I was ready to go full tilt again.

By November, it seemed the Lord spoke to my heart that He was going to take me down to nothing, but would raise me up again to new life, much like Jesus rose from the dead. I questioned that this was from the Lord, as I did not understand what this could possibly mean. I thought that I had been through enough! This seemed so ominous and frightening.

The shortness of breath continued on, getting worse and worse. It got to the point where I could not even attempt to go upstairs at the church; I had to use the elevator. Week after week, I led the praise and worship at the church, as I believed the Lord wanted me to do. There were times it was difficult to even make it through a phrase of a song because of the shortness of breath. But God was always faithful to me, and His anointing never failed to be upon me as I led the praise and worship.

On November 16, 2000, I had my first mammogram since the breast cancer was discovered. My radiologist examined me. I explained to him the shortness of breath and lack of energy I had been experiencing. I was so weary of not feeling well. He ascertained that I had inflammation in the chest wall. He prescribed Naproxen to alleviate that inflammation.

The next day, I had a scheduled appointment with my primary physician. With care, he asked me the pointed question, "How are you mentally handling the breast cancer?" Almost immediately, I started crying. He recommended that I begin taking Zoloft to help me deal with the tumultuous changes occurring in my life. He said typically cancer patients are on Zoloft for six months to a year, helping them to cope with life. I began taking the Naproxen and Zoloft on Friday night, November 17.

Within twenty-four hours, it appeared that I had been plagued with an all-out case of arthritis over my entire body. Joints began to ache. It first started in my knees. Next, I noticed my jaw hurting. My upper arms began to hurt; only that didn't seem to be in the joints. I thank God it never extended to my hips or neck, two areas in my body that were already weak due to previous accidents. Every day it seemed that another joint would begin to erupt with pain. *I had pain twenty-four hours a day.* Nothing I did would dismiss the pain.

I could not handle giving love and affection to our daughters. This was difficult for the girls to understand. They wanted and needed their mommy. This was painful not only physically, but emotionally as well. I was concerned for the effect this would have on the girls' psyches. Ken had to spend extra time giving them love and affection. This had to suffice, but it was not the same as hugs and cuddles from their mother.

I contacted each of the physicians who had me under their care. Each one was baffled by this occurrence. After all, I was taking medication that should have relieved pain in the joints, not cause it. I even checked with my pharmacist, Henry, who was Linda's husband, and knew me well as friends do. He could not figure this out either. His recommendation was to take extra-strength Tylenol in between the Naproxen. This helped to manage the pain, but I still dealt with pain continuously.

The only conclusion we discerned for this extreme reaction was an attack of Satan. The enemy of my soul wanted to snuff out my life altogether and stop me from ministering to people. There was no other logical explanation at the time.

Because of the pain, I grew weaker. I could no longer do much around the house. I would attempt to put clean sheets on the bed, but I could not handle the enormous amount of pain surging through my body. Ken helped me with the housework. He did not need this extra concern at home; he was still making the necessary adjustments of learning a new job and industry.

Our sixth wedding anniversary was Tuesday, November 21. How could we celebrate? We celebrated our love for each other in spite of the present circumstances. We were thankful to be together and always enjoyed our times of aloneness, whenever we could manage that to happen.

The lowest peak for me came the next night, the Wednesday night before Thanksgiving. We had to change our Thanksgiving plans to go to Oshkosh, Wisconsin, where Jerry and Laura (one of Ken's brothers and his wife) live. I had fought the pain for so long and with people around me all the time. I just needed and wanted some time to myself where I didn't have to pretend to feel better than I did. I stayed home from church while Ken and the girls went. That night as I lay on the sofa attempting to watch TV and relax, I found it difficult to concentrate. I was in so much pain just lying there without even moving! The covers felt very heavy, and it actually hurt to have them over me.

When Ken and the girls came home from church, I attempted to get up from the sofa to help him put the girls to bed. It took a while to figure out how to maneuver my body from the sofa with the least amount of pain. My mind drifted back to the days of being pregnant. I had to learn how to remove myself from the sofa. At least back then, I had gracefully managed my pregnant body from the sofa. This was totally different. It was impossible. All I could do was grin and bear the pain. I had always told myself to smile no matter how much pain I was in. Even that resolve was now being tested.

As the pain continued to spread each day, it went to the elbows, the hands, and the feet. My ankles became swollen. My left arm would go numb in the night, and the stinging and burning sensations seemed unbearable. I would lie awake for a while until it settled down again. There was nothing I could do to relieve the discomfort. This went on, night after night. I was losing sleep every night due to the pain. I have always preferred sleeping on my left side, but that position only intensified the pain. I would attempt to sleep on my right side or my back. Getting on my right side was a real trick, because that was the arm that would not work. My right arm would experience excruciating pain if I attempted to raise it. Even through the pain, Ken and I would laugh. It all seemed so ridiculous! I felt like such an invalid.

Getting in and out of bed was tedious as well. I didn't realize the muscles involved in getting around until I lost the ability to do the simplest things. As the pain continued to be almost more than I could take, I wondered if I would lose my mind. My body was writhing in pain, night after night. I did not know what was going to happen to me. Would I have to enter a nursing home facility? How much longer could Ken care for me? With Ken now employed and working full time, with an additional hour on the road to and from work, I was left at home to care for our daughters. I would sometimes let out an excruciating "ouch" and the girls wondered if their mommy was all right. I regularly explained to them I hurt badly.

All the while, I held on to Jesus with everything in me. I knew what the Lord had spoken to me. I knew this was what He was referring to when He said He would take me down to nothing. I was there. I felt lower than a lizard's lung. Still, I had hope in the deep recesses of my mind, knowing that God would raise me up again like He had done for His Son, Jesus. It took everything within me to hold on to Jesus, believing He would see me through this difficulty. I began to think of people I knew or had known in my life who suffered continual pain. Empathy rose inside of me for people that hurt with pain.

After suffering with this joint pain for two weeks, I began to notice some improvement. The shortness of breath and the other symptoms of the inflammation in the chest wall were gone! I was most grateful for progress of any kind! I was still tolerating the joint pain and not understanding why I had to suffer so much. After all, the radiation treatments were completed. I was more than ready to get on with my life. It was time, so I thought.

I was left with no explanation with the joint pain. It wasn't until years later medical studies revealed Naproxen combined with Zoloft could cause this very side effect.

Gradually, very gradually, with each day growing closer to Christmas, the joint pain improved a little. It was indeed strange I had to go through this, but it taught me what only pain can teach a person. Some of my old attitudes of not having compassion for people in hurting situations vanished as I endured the pain. I realized I needed to see people the way Christ sees them. This did not mean making sport of their shortcomings, no matter what they were.

It took a while for my dexterity to return to normal. At least I was able to be my bubbly self at church again and the congregation was extremely elated. It was still a little tender to get down on my knees. On the outer edges of my feet, it still hurt at times. The palm side by the left thumb still hurt. The right arm continued to hurt upon being raised, but at least some movement was now possible. At night when I got tired, my whole body would go into a cramping mode. I knew to either fall asleep or be miserable. Another thing I noticed when I got extremely tired, like on Sunday nights, I inwardly shook. That was very disconcerting to me, but relaxing seemed to be the only remedy.

I was terribly wound up during this time. This bothered me, but considering what my body had been through, it seemed logical. I just knew that I had to get better, and I tried to do everything I knew to do. I asked the Lord, begging Him, to please help me get better, as I had had enough to deal with this year. At least I was now feeling enough better that I could get my mind off myself and on others who needed ministering. I believed that by redirecting my energy to meeting others' needs, I would get the total healing I needed.

It had been a very dark place. It had been a time of extreme loneliness. I felt like I was being alienated from God and people.

As the year came to a close, I reflected on the year and what God had taught me in and through my life. I was amazed by the year as a whole and God's faithfulness to Ken, the girls, and me. Through this last round of pain, I had finally realized it was all about dying to self. That's what was meant by taking me down to nothing. As Christ humbled himself by coming to this earth and dying on a cruel cross, so I must humble myself and die daily to the temptations around me.

The first week of January 2001 ushered in the death of my 101-year-old grandmother. She was the last of my grandparents to die. Even though I had been ready for her death for years, as her quality of life had diminished over the last few years, I had entertained the thought that perhaps she was simply too stubborn to die.

When asked by my mother and aunt to perform her funeral, I willingly accepted this awesome privilege. I knew my grandma, her good points and bad points. Grandma had a lot of spunk and determination that I knew I had inherited from her. She was a prayer warrior. She told me years before that she prayed for each one of her grandchildren every morning.

It was difficult on my mother to lose her mother, even at her age. I needed to minister to my mother at this time. This took extra time and energy outside of my normal activities of church and home.

A few weeks after my grandmother's funeral, I realized I finally felt like my old self again. I felt free to get on with my life. What a relief this was: breast cancer was behind me—at long last—after nine months!

CHAPTER SIX

I am overwhelmed with joy in the Lord my God!
For he has dressed me with the clothing of salva-
tion and draped me in a robe of righteousness.

Isaiah 61:10

Spring was just around the corner. The grass
was beginning to turn green; buds were coming on the
trees. This was my favorite time of year. It could not
be more appropriate for the dead of winter to vanish
and the newness of spring to become reality. Certainly,
I had been through a winter season in my life, and
now I was experiencing the fullness of life in all its
magnificence.

I had some catching up to do with my two little girls.
They were always a part of the process, yet I felt I had
disturbed their toddler years. Perhaps the girls could
use this lesson in their lives and become more compassionate people as a result of our journey through breast
cancer. Is this what it would teach our daughters? I certainly did not want it to teach them fear.

I had some catching up to do with my husband too. Being seven years older than him, would he have married me, had he known that I would have such health problems? If I had only been younger than him, perhaps I would have been a healthier woman. Yet I knew that I should not be second-guessing myself. It was quite clear to Ken and me that God had brought us together, as this has never been an issue in our marriage. Our lives had been bonded in such a supernatural way through our early years of marriage. Most marriages have their own unique struggles. It just seemed we had more than our share. This trying time did not tear us apart. Spending time talking and sharing our deepest thoughts, our love for each other only grew stronger. We were in this together, and with God's help and strength, we would carry on with the Lord's work.

I gave myself permission to enjoy life again. I had started a ladies' Bible study in the fall, and a camaraderie among the women had already taken place. I continued with the choir and the Easter musical preparation. My ministry at the church was in full force, and I was a happy camper! I loved working for the Lord. It brought such joy and fulfillment to my life.

During this time, an amazing occurrence took place in the area of emotional healing. The breast cancer had been symbolic in a physical sense of what I was dealing with emotionally. We all have cancer in our bodies, whether we realize it or not. It comes in many different forms, but it is there trying to eat away the good cells. This emotional healing came in bits and pieces. It was a lengthy process, but ultimately worth all the angst and energy.

Emotional healing reminded me of a physical sickness. The stomach churns and aches and groans with discomfort. There is something in the stomach that is causing the problem. There is only one solution: vomit up the offending matter. Only then can you know what caused this discomfort. It was a similar process in an emotional sense. Something had been bothering me for a long time, and now, at long last, I had "vomited up" the discomfort. Then came relief. I had been emotionally freed and made well.

My life's deepest disappointments and painful memories had been long buried, leaving grave emotional scars. Dealing with the breast cancer had caused me to turn inward, dredging up the hurts of the past in full measure. I was already dealing with so much, and now I was forced to revisit and analyze several past personal relationships. I realized I needed more than physical healing; I needed emotional healing if I was to move forward. I became aware of several unresolved issues from my past that needed to be dealt with. It was, to say the least, an unpleasant process as I began examining situations involving people from my past.

Over several months, I took a series of one-day road trips with Linda, and we talked and talked. Our friendship was relatively new, and there should have been little baggage, but because of hurts at the hands of old friends, our friendship was suffering. Linda would question me about the way I reacted to certain things, treating her as though she would desert the friendship if I acted up. I had experienced many relationships that seemed to want too much from me while giving back too little. It seemed all too often my own opinions were ignored or discounted. If I pressed with my opinions, I was either put down or the friendship ended.

As far back as I can remember, my childhood has left me with the feeling that I did not quite belong. This feeling carried over from home to school. I had just graduated from high school when a female cousin I was particularly close with suddenly died after a two-week bout of herpes encephalitis. In my grief, I turned to my pastor's wife. A bond had just started to form when she suddenly left her husband for another man. Another connection was lost, and I was very confused. Over and over, I seemed to allow myself to become close to someone only to lose him or her through death or other circumstances.

As a young adult, I had a dear friend who accompanied me through the long and painful process of recovering from injuries incurred in an automobile accident. I had been hit by a drunk driver. My problems were financial as well as physical, and a long court battle ensued. The day finally came when the trial was over, and suddenly the friendship ended. The only explanation she offered was that she was angry because I had not asked her to help me pick out my new living room furnishings. What kind of excuse was that for ending a friendship? I will never know what was behind the dissolution of our relationship.

Yet another girlfriend was so dear to me. We did not let miles that separated us physically dilute our affection for one another. We would talk for hours, discussing and solving our problems. The friendship was mutually therapeutic, or so I thought. After an extended time of not hearing from her, I became concerned. I learned from her cousin that my dear friend had committed suicide while on sabbatical with her husband in England. I was devastated at this new and senseless loss.

My chosen career as a music pastor was taking me down a new path filled with new emotional challenges. One of the first churches where I served as a staff pastor was led by a man who had severe anger management issues. With little or no provocation, he would explode, spewing verbal venom, and most often I was the target for his tirades. He basically found me to his dislike because I was female and an unmarried female at that. He was often most explicit in his enumeration of about all my physical and professional shortfalls. I have never been able to tolerate being yelled at because of a childhood filled with my mother's frequent outbursts. As a child, my escape was going to the piano and practicing until the storm had passed. As an adult, my only refuge was hiding in the ladies' room at the church. I felt so isolated. This pastor was very careful to schedule these regular outbursts when there were no other witnesses to hear him berate me.

After too much of this abuse, I tendered my resignation. The scars of his negativity left me with serious doubts about my ability to serve in the capacity of music pastor. I had been effectively beaten down. The next senior pastor under which I served had many of the same personality traits as the last one. He was not abusive, but I found myself allowing my bad experience to affect my working relationship with him. He was actually a very good man, but I could not get beyond what had occurred in my former position. There was no trust or professional cohesiveness between us, and this resulted in a very poor working relationship. Once again, I felt overwhelmed by failure and disappointment in myself and those I had trusted.

A new friend became very important to me. She was such a dear friend, but neither of us knew how to set time boundaries with one other. It soon became an unhealthy and obsessive relationship. When my family moved to Iowa and distance should have tempered the intensity of the relationship, she became very needy. I had made a new life for me and my family. There was a new job, new responsibilities, and two small children, as well as a husband, needing my constant attention. It became necessary to ask her to stop calling me so frequently. This proved too difficult and the friendship ended. We were eventually able to communicate on occasion, and I felt the rift had been mended.

It has been an exhilarating feeling to be set free from the past. I have unearthed and dealt with so many deeply entrenched hurts and I am now experiencing the wonderful liberty of a true emotional healing. The sky is the limit when a person has been emotionally set free through Christ and His sacrifice on Calvary. There were people I needed to forgive, and I wrote letters to each one asking for their forgiveness. I received their absolution, and they asked me for mine, which I gave gladly. I had put to rest the past, and it had lost the power to dictate my future. Forgiveness brought closure and a sweet freedom. It no longer mattered how people treated me. I knew I was responsible for my own reactions. I knew that regardless of what people said or did, my heavenly Father loved me. He held me in His loving arms. All I had to do was run to Him.

As a young girl, at times I would reach out my hand, imagining I was holding Jesus's hand when I felt afraid or alone. Imaginary handholding was no longer enough. As a grownup, I needed to be held in my heavenly Father's infinite arms. I longed to know and feel His love for me. I was never disappointed by this love, ever constant and true.

When God's love permeates your very being, fear is dispelled. God's love is able to eradicate the worst fear. Through truly experiencing His love, fear is replaced by peace. As prayer and communion with the Lord grows, perfect love and peace infuse one's being.

We can find this sweet place in Him, but life still happens. We don't stay in our heavenly Father's loving arms. We return to the everyday of life and return to doing things our own way. We get comfortable and complacent in our daily routine, thinking all is well in our little world once more.

Spring passed all too quickly and summer was upon us. I was looking forward to enjoying this summer with everything in me. The summer instead proved to be quite hectic. On top of that, I began to experience discomfort and pain in my lower abdomen. I did not know why I was having such pain. A part of me could not help but wonder if it was cancer related. After all, having cancer changes everything. Any ache or pain I experienced would always raise the question in the back of my mind: am I dealing with cancer again? This continued for several weeks as summer bowed its head.

By Friday, September 14, 2001, I had made an appointment with my surgeon. With my oncologist and my surgeon's recommendations, a hysterectomy was scheduled. Both physicians knew the Tamoxifen would work more effectively in my body to prevent further breast cancer if the ovaries were removed. My oncologist had informed me that estrogen was my body's enemy, as that had been the culprit of breast cancer in the first place. Any form of removing estrogen from my body was beneficial to me not getting breast cancer again. There was also the possibility of developing uterine cancer since my mother had it.

Not even a year and a half had passed since the initial breast cancer was discovered and now I was scheduled for a hysterectomy. I knew there would be pros and cons to this surgery, yet I knew it was the right decision. I could not continue enduring the pain in my abdomen.

Once again, it was difficult letting everyone know that I would have a hysterectomy. It was a common surgery among women. As a result of this, I received plenty of unsolicited advice. My mother had a hysterectomy, and because of her brush with death at that time, a lingering fear came to me in her remembered words. On learning of my impending surgery, she had said to me, "Karen, your girls and Ken need you very much, but your dad and I need you also." I had no fear of dying at this time. Perhaps my mother was willing me to live. I had my own strength and a determination to live was rooted deeply inside of me. I wanted to live!

I was tired of surgeries and prayed this would be my last. After all, I had endured my share of surgeries. Looking back to right after Mackenzie was born, I recalled the appendectomy I had. Ken and I had gotten up around four o'clock in the morning to feed Mackenzie. I was overcome by pain in the lower right side of my abdomen. We immediately thought it was appendicitis. We called friends to come and stay with the girls. Ken took me to the hospital.

When the hospital personnel greet you with familiarity, it can only be a bad sign! I had given birth to Mackenzie only thirteen days before. The usual blood tests were taken, and the prognosis of appendicitis was quickly made. My appendix was removed laparoscopically. However, the pathology report showed the appendix was not the problem. It was a good appendix. It turned out I had a post-natal uterine infection. A round of antibiotics was given to treat this. Now here I was, not only recovering from childbirth, but surgery as well. This was in October of 1998.

I was scheduled for a hysterectomy on Tuesday, September 18, 2001. It had been determined I had a cyst on one of my ovaries. During the surgery, the surgeon discovered that the cyst had ruptured. Two days later, the pathology report came back: no cancer! Ken and I were not only relieved, but our hearts were grateful to the Lord for His hand upon me.

When I awoke in the recovery room from the anesthesia, the first thing I noticed was the pain I had been suffering was totally gone. I felt like a person with a new lease on life. By Thursday night, Ken told me he had not seen that certain grin on my face for several years. This surgery over, I felt carefree for the first time in a long time. I could not believe how good I felt!

The pain from the incision caused me minimal discomfort. I was rejoicing in the newness of life I was now experiencing!

I was dismissed from the hospital by Friday afternoon, September 21. Ken's parents had arrived to spend a few days helping us around the house. It was nice to have the much-needed assistance. It was indeed special to have Mom and Dad Norton here for Mackenzie's third birthday on September 24. We invited family on my side as well for the birthday celebration. Mackenzie was born on my parents' anniversary and forevermore was my present to them.

Healing comes more slowly to an impatient person. When the surgeon told me it would take six weeks to heal, he was not joking. No matter how much willpower I possessed, I could not move the healing process along more quickly. Fortunately, we had bought two recliners in May that would now be critical for getting the recuperative sleep I so desperately needed. I slept each night for several weeks in my recliner. It was most uncomfortable attempting to sleep in bed. If I tried stretching out in bed, it was painful around the incision area. If I moved around in bed, it was painful. If Ken moved around in bed, it was painful. I was more stationary in my recliner, making it easier to sleep.

While I was recuperating, the Lord was working on me. It was a humbling experience to have people from the church do our family's laundry. Because I didn't have the energy to deal with it, the idea didn't bother me that much. That surprised the "private Karen" that I knew. I was so grateful for the prayers going up to heaven on our family's behalf, but the physical works did not go unappreciated either. Meals were brought in. People from the church would come to play with and care for our girls.

Allison and Mackenzie were fascinated by their mommy's incision. They watched me like a hawk as I grimaced with the pain from the surgery. But I was happy and joyful. I felt like a new person.

I was very anxious to get on with my life. The six weeks of recovery passed quickly as it would for any mother of toddlers. I was on my way to settling in again with the church work that I had missed dearly. I had behaved myself during those six weeks and was able to work once again.

Christmas musical preparations were before me. Life became hectic once again. Finding time to have fun and do some Christmas shopping, Linda and I took a day off. Ken took a day off from his job to stay with the girls. At long last, it was good to get out. There is something therapeutic about shopping.

Linda and I were having a great time shopping. Traffic was typically busy for December. Without warning, we were involved in an automobile accident. Sandwiched between two vans, I saw it coming in my rearview mirror. I prayed a quick, "Dear Lord, help us!" under my breath. It could have done more damage, but the Lord was gracious to us. We were so thankful the girls were not with us. Damage was done to the front and rear of our combination SUV and minivan, totaling 4,900 dollars. Linda and I suffered whiplash injuries.

Over the next nine months to a year, I found myself visiting my chiropractor regularly. For one month, I suffered a headache *every single day*. This ailment cut into the productivity and creativity necessary for my position as music pastor. My responsibilities of wife and mother at home were compromised as well.

I found myself bitter. Again, my joy was taken from me by this latest accident. I did not want to suffer through another healing process. Life seemed to be one time of healing after another. This is not what I wanted from life. I wanted to be emptied of myself and focus on other people, ministering to their needs. What I did not realize was the more I experienced the process of pain, suffering, and healing, the more compassion I was developing for other people. The Lord was once again using my pain to teach me something of greater significance.

After so many consecutive negative things happen, it becomes obvious to a Christian that there is an enemy, and he is waging war with us. He was long ago defeated when Jesus rose from the dead. The victory is ours through Jesus! Though we are victorious, we still suffer in this life. A normal person does not want to suffer. This is where the battle lies.

CHAPTER SEVEN

I am always overwhelmed with a desire for your
regulations.

Psalm 119:20

If I had any personal goals or desires for the year
2002, it would be no more surgeries in my life. I continued to deal with the pain and agony of recovering
from the automobile accident, and I was doing fairly
well by the time summer was in full force.

Determined to make this summer a summer to
remember, I strove to be an entertaining mother. This
was the last summer before our firstborn, Allison Grace,
would start kindergarten. Even before the girls were
born, I wanted to be the best mother these girls could
have. How I had longed to be a mother for so many
years! These were their formative years. I vowed not
to let one moment of one day pass without cherishing
them. Days were spent with regular trips to local parks,
traveling to a large zoo and spending the day there,
and of course, a family vacation before school began. I

juggled my job as activities director for the home while maintaining my part-time position as music pastor at the church. I loved every minute of it!

The senior pastor had hired a delightful children's pastor in her twenties who reminded me of myself at that age. We became fast friends. Allison and Mackenzie enjoyed their new children's pastor. It was nice for the girls to establish a new relationship with their very own children's pastor.

Summer ended all too quickly. Allison must start kindergarten. The first day was traumatic on daughter and mother alike. Tears punctuated the moment of separation as this new life's chapter opened and another closed. My little girl, my firstborn daughter, was about to begin a new journey.

Fortunately, the Christian school in which we had Allison enrolled was across the street from the church. With Allison in school, I could put in regular part-time office hours. Allison went to school three days a week, all day, on Mondays, Wednesdays, and Fridays. Mackenzie would entertain herself by coloring or playing with toys while I worked at the church. This was beneficial to establishing better working relationships with the staff at the church as well as being more productive at the church and at home. I would work at the church while Allison was in school. This proved a soothing balm for the ache of separation.

As school gradually became a routine in the Norton household, a change was noted in Mackenzie. At first, Ken and I thought she was grieving the loss of her sister as a daily playmate. After all, Mackenzie had only known life with Allison up to this point. It was evident she not only loved her older sister, but looked up to her and wanted to do everything Allison did.

Still, something was amiss with Mackenzie. People in the church, especially her Sunday school teachers, could tell something was wrong. When we named our younger daughter Mackenzie Joy, we had no idea that joy would be her very personality. She was always bright-eyed and happy. But these days Mackenzie was anything but happy. Her eyes grew dark and clouded. She began to speak of her stomach hurting her on a daily basis.

Mackenzie had been born with an abdominal hernia above the navel. At the time of her birth, our pediatrician indicated this would have to be surgically corrected at some time in the future. This was not the usual umbilical hernia that most babies outgrow. There was no need to operate on Mackenzie until it became a problem to her. It was obvious the time had come!

We took Mackenzie to our pediatrician, who, in turn, recommended a children's surgeon in a nearby city. The problem was pretty straightforward as was the solution. Surgery was inevitable. The incision would be inside the navel, so a visible scar would never be seen.

On October 24, 2002, the time for her surgery came very early. In fact, Allison spent the night at Linda and Henry's house where we knew she would be in good hands. This was Mackenzie's day, and our complete focus and attention were on her and her needs. Ken took off work and away we went, some forty miles to the children's hospital. It was an outpatient procedure, so we would bring Mackenzie home with us after a time of recovery.

The most difficult part was when the nurse took Mackenzie away for the surgical prep. I held tightly to Ken, as I watched our daughter's frightened face disappear through the doors. I had to be brave and tell Mackenzie everything was going to be okay. I knew she would be okay. There's just something about watching your child in so much pain and not being able to do anything about it.

When Mackenzie came out of surgery and had some time in recovery, she was brought back to Ken and me. She wanted me to hold her, which I gladly did. She held on tightly to me, unsure of what was going on. After the appropriate time had passed, we were dismissed from the hospital and headed home.

After picking up Allison at Linda's house, we went home, reunited as a family. After being home a few minutes, Ken and I ventured into the girls' bedroom to find Mackenzie jumping freely on their bed! Her impish smile had returned! We didn't even scold her for jumping on the bed, as we were truly blessed to have our younger daughter back to normal again!

The obvious change in Mackenzie was noticed among church members, family, and friends. Everyone joined us with elation over Mackenzie's recovery. She had returned to her joyful self. We may never know how long she had silently been suffering with this ailment. Praise God, it was over now.

With the closing of 2002, we received the news that our youth pastor and his wife were leaving us to pastor a church in another state. This would be an adjustment for the church, as a big void would have to be filled.

Changes are always a challenge. At times, we may think we are ready for a change, only to realize we are flirting with the-grass-is-greener-on-the-other-side mentality. Some of us desire change to avoid boredom. As a young girl, I recalled my mother telling me one time, "Karen, I have never seen a more changeable person than you!" She knew how I longed for change, never remaining the same. I wanted life to be fresh and new each and every day.

Over the years and due to circumstances in my life, I had changed. Still, the drive and desire for progress lingered inside of me.

CHAPTER EIGHT

I think of God, and I moan, overwhelmed with longing for his help.

Psalm 77:3

It seemed that life was going smoothly. It was now 2003, and good things were starting to happen. Being in the ministry always brought challenges, but it was always a joy to serve people. I loved watching people grow and develop in the Lord.

There are times we think that things will stay the same and our present circumstances will never change. Good or bad, we accept life as it is. Then comes the unexpected and our world begins to unravel. At first, we may not even recognize what is happening.

For years, Ken and I had discussed my having a breast reduction. I was healed from my previous surgeries, and someone mentioned to me that it might be a good idea to look into having it done. The time seemed right for this procedure. Somehow, we knew in our spirits that now was the time to pursue this surgery.

I contacted my oncologist to make sure this was not a problem after having breast cancer. He assured me it would not be a problem and recommended a plastic surgeon he knew. I went to this plastic surgeon in April 2003. We discussed the possibility of having the breast reduction. Given my history of breast cancer, the location of my scar, and the radiation treatments, this plastic surgeon wanted some time before making a decision to operate on me. I appreciated his professional approach and decided to allow him the time he needed to review my records.

A week later, I returned to the plastic surgeon. After weighing the pros and cons, he believed it to be too risky for him to perform the breast reduction. He recommended I see the plastic surgeon at the university hospital, who was more specialized in this overall procedure. Instead of forty miles away, we would travel approximately eighty miles to the University of Iowa Hospital.

My first office consultation with this new plastic surgeon was in June. This was nothing new or different for this doctor. He had seen cases like mine and performed many breast reductions on women with histories similar to mine. He did give me the rehearsed speech about the worst-case scenario of possible things that could go awry with this procedure. However, he did not encounter any red flags. The surgery was scheduled. "Scheduled" meant a few months away, however. I was anxious and impatient, wanting to get this latest surgery behind me. The breast reduction surgery was scheduled for September 30.

Things at the church had become extremely strenuous. Upon much prayer, our delightful children's pastor decided to resign. The senior pastor and I now were the only pastors on board. We had gone from four pastors down to two in just a few months' time. Much of the summer lay ahead of us. There was camp to think about and getting young people to and from their designated camps. The load of responsibility became quite demanding for my part-time position as music pastor. We were uncertain of the future of the church and finding suitable pastoral staff members. The church desperately needed a youth pastor and a children's pastor.

The senior pastor and his wife took their yearly two-week vacation in July. I became the sole pastor for the church during this time. Thankfully, there were no funerals to be conducted while they were away!

It is difficult to discern when it is time for a pastor to move on from a church. There was a knowing in the spirits of the senior pastor and his wife that their time at this church was ending. Likewise, Ken and I felt a release in our spirits and knew the time had come to resign. It was time to move on. We believed it was in the church's best interest to have a clean slate and start with a new pastoral staff. This would enable the church of two hundred people to press on with the fresh vision that a new senior pastor would bring.

Our summer vacation came in August before Allison started school. It would be a soul-searching, thought-provoking time for earnest prayer kind of vacation. We knew that upon returning home I would be resigning from the church as music pastor. What did the Lord have for us next? Where would be the next place that the Lord would call us to minister?

We spent a glorious family vacation in Colorado. This was the girls' and my first visit to the Rocky Mountains. What a breathtaking view of God's wonders, His mountains! We managed to spend a few days in the home of one of my dearest friends from Bible college. After all these years, being able to reminisce and get to know each other's husbands and children was a fun time. This vacation was off to a great start. We knew it was going to be a wonderful vacation, certainly a much-needed one. We experienced all forms of weather, from snow and sleet in the mountains to the hot and dry desert air of the Great Sand Dunes. Camping was an adventure given the variety of weather conditions. We were able to find the added mental and emotional strength we needed for what lay ahead of us when we returned home. We spent our last Sunday at an Assemblies of God church where the services were excellent, and the pastor and his wife were most hospitable. We were able to share with peers what we were experiencing back home. We knew these newfound friends would keep us in their prayers.

We had resigned on August 24, with our last Sunday being September 21. Allison had begun the first grade at the Christian school on August 25. It was tentative as to how long Allison would continue at this school, but we had to proceed.

I sent out résumés, grasping for God's direction for my ministry and for our family.

In spite of my knowing in my spirit our time was ended at the church, it still hit me like a death in the family. There was so much unknowing of what the future held for our family. We had struggled to gain a foothold here in this community with Ken's lack of employment nearly five years earlier. Now it was time to move on to wherever the Lord would have us to go. Still, there was an uneasiness in my spirit. I sensed we would be detained from future ministry. I did not relish the thought of this. I tried telling myself I was being negative and everything would work out for our good. Yet I continued to wrestle with this nagging uneasiness in my spirit.

CHAPTER NINE

Deeper and deeper I sink into the mire; I can't find a foothold. I am in deep water, and the floods overwhelm me.

Psalm 69:2

Though still numb from resigning my music pastor position at the church, I pressed forward in anticipation of the breast reduction. My surgery was less than two weeks away.

The church had sent us off with a fabulous reception the last Sunday night following the evening service. So much love and sentiment was shared by the people at that time. Our family had truly been blessed by a loving congregation over the last five years.

Our lives were in God's hands. We did not know what He had in store for us, but we remained hopeful. A deep longing stirred inside of us as we pursued God's will for our lives.

Ken and I believed it was imperative to communicate with our daughters what was going on in our lives. We did not know how much longer we would live here. The future looked uncertain for us remaining in our current home. Poor Allison would go to school each day, wondering how much longer she would be with her friends in first grade, with her lovely teacher who seemed to understand Allison so well right from the start. Mackenzie was content being her mommy's shadow and coloring pictures for hours on end.

I quickly learned my support system was dwindling. No longer having the ladies' Bible study at the church was an enormous emotional loss. I had had between twelve to fifteen ladies in my close-knit circle with the choir and the Bible study group. It was now time for them to move on. Another choir director was appointed. Another Bible study leader stepped into position. I knew all this had to happen, but why weren't our lives moving on?

This was only the beginning of our latest round of testing.

Ken took time off from work to be with me for the breast reduction surgery. I had to be in the hospital overnight for this procedure. My parents willingly came to our home to tend to the girls' needs. Allison needed to be taken to school and picked up each day. Mackenzie became close to her grandpa, as they spent time together assembling jigsaw puzzles.

Step one for the breast reduction procedure was to be marked up with a magic marker the day before surgery. That evening, Ken and I discussed a variety of additional markings we could have inserted to make things even more interesting, but decided to behave ourselves instead.

As the plastic surgeon visited with us one last time before the procedure, he asked the sixty-million-dollar question, "What do we do if we discover cancer while performing the operation?" He caught me off guard with this question.

I told him to remove the cancer. I did not want it left inside of me to grow. I just could not imagine that I had any more cancer, as I knew my prognosis was excellent.

I walked away from the plastic surgeon's office a little shook up. Cancer? How dare he mention the C word to me! I had served my time, I knew the experience, and I was not going there again!

This conversation with the plastic surgeon had given Ken and me pause. We drove around the area and later had a nice dinner on the eve of the surgery. We had secured a hotel room for the night, as the distance from home coupled with the early surgical time made it easier to stay in town. Ken and I spent this quality time together to share concerns and fears about the doctor's pointed question. We were able to calmly discuss the subject during this time.

Lying in bed that night, however, I became apprehensive. I tried telling myself it was silly to worry. After all, I was having a breast reduction! I was taking a load off my shoulders and back. I could not imagine what it would feel like. How exciting to be able to have this surgery! It had been in the works for about six months. Years earlier, Ken and I had discussed the possibility, but now it was becoming a reality. This was actually a surgery that I *wanted*. That, in itself, was truly amazing. I had entertained doubts that I was becoming addicted to surgeries, thinking it was necessary to have them frequently. I knew this was absurd. Nevertheless, I tossed and turned that night, awaiting the surgery and wondering how it would change my life.

The next morning as we prepared for the surgery, the sun was shining brightly on this beautiful fall day, the last day of September. It seemed unusual not to have a pastor or friend along with Ken and me. We were alone in a strange town, experiencing this surgery together. I knew this was how it was meant to be. It was best to do it this way.

I had shared with some friends and family members what we were about to do. We received responses both in favor and against our decision. Perhaps it took courage on my part to even want to make this change. I was not unhappy with the way God had made me. I truly believed Psalm 139:13–14: "You made all the delicate, inner parts of my body and knit me together in my mother's womb. Thank you for making me so wonderfully complex! Your workmanship is marvelous—how well I know it."

Sustained by my faith, I found the courage I needed for the time. Hand in hand, Ken and I walked together into the hospital. I pushed aside the apprehensive feelings I had wrestled with during the long night. I was excited for this surgery to take place! I would look like a different person with a reduced bust.

A few hours later I woke from surgery, feeling like a tremendous burden had been taken off my shoulders. My old breasts were gone! No more droopy, saggy, and cumbersome breasts, I now had the perfect-sized breasts on my body! The pain from the surgery was so minimal. The incisions looked like anchors to a ship, all but invisible. The nipples had also been reduced in size in accordance to the new size of the breasts.

To say that I was flying high after this surgery would be an understatement. I had to stay in the hospital overnight but then got to return home. Ken had to go back to work, so my friend June was able to pick me up and drive me home. June and Linda were the two friends that remained close to me. At this time, Linda was preparing for open-heart surgery after months of not feeling well.

I was so thankful that June could take me home. She, like Linda, had a way about her that made me feel comfortable with myself, and I always knew my confidences were well kept. I had to ride in the car with a pillow on my front because of a tiny amount of pain. The eighty-two-mile ride home went quickly by as June and I yakked our way home. We marveled at the Lord allowing me this luxury of having my breasts reduced. I couldn't help but remark on how little pain I had. I was so very thankful for that.

I was scheduled to see the plastic surgeon again in five days for a follow-up visit. Other than that, I was home free! I was enjoying a new life with my now perfect-sized breasts! I wondered what it would be like to once again be in front of a congregation ministering.

So very little pain after the surgery made this a real festive time in more ways than one. I came home to our daughters, Allison (now six years old) and Mackenzie (now five years old), all wide-eyed and full of questions as to what had happened to their mommy's boobies! I took the time to explain to them that I had surgery to take away some of Mommy's boobies because I had too much and it was causing me a lot of shoulder and back pain. They were very attentive and fascinated by all I had to say.

The next five days went quickly, and June was able to take me back for my follow-up appointment, since I had not been released yet to drive. I was so very thankful that she could take the time to do this. It meant so much to me. Ken had to work, and the girls were being taken care of.

The plastic surgeon examined me, telling me everything looked great. He could tell by my facial expression that I was a happy camper with my new breasts. I thanked him over and over for performing this operation on me.

He then asked me if I had seen the pathology report. I told him I had not. He looked through my files and could not find it. He excused himself out of the examination room to hunt down the information. Seconds turned into minutes, and the minutes were long. June and I talked, but I became apprehensive. I could not imagine what was taking so long. Everything had gone like clockwork.

Suddenly, the plastic surgeon came back into the room. "Mrs. Norton, I'm afraid I have some terrible news for you," he said. I thought he surely must be joking, but his voice revealed otherwise.

"What is it?"

"I am so sorry, but the pathology report shows there is cancer in both breasts."

While my head spun from this horrific blow, he went on to explain to me the pathology report indicated the pathologists had dissected and cut every which way looking for cancer since I had a past history of breast cancer. They had already prepared extra specimens, but they decided to look one last time from a different angle. It was then they found the cancer in both breasts!

CHAPTER TEN

When calamity overtakes you like a storm, when disaster engulfs you like a cyclone, and anguish and distress overwhelm you.

Proverbs 1:27

"You will need to notify your oncologist of this prognosis of breast cancer. Would you like for us to do this for you?" the plastic surgeon asked. Trying to hold myself together, I struggled to absorb this news of breast cancer once again. I thanked the doctor for his offer to notify my oncologist. This was all in God's plan. Somehow, it had to be God's plan even though at the moment I could not believe what I was hearing. I was so thankful June was with me. I did not need to hear this news by myself and then drive the distance home. I was also grateful that the pathologists had been so thorough in dissecting the breast tissue. There was no doubt in my mind what I was facing.

Upon leaving the university hospital campus, I called Ken on my cell phone. Oh, how I hated making that call to my husband, who had already gone down this road with me once and now had to make the journey with me once again. There was no easy way to break the news, so I blurted it out. His response was, "Oh, no!" He knew the only way to handle it was with the Lord's help and strength. This was not the path of our choosing, but for reasons known only to Him, God was using this recurring cancer to mold us further into the character and likeness of His Son, Jesus.

As June and I traveled back home, I was on my cell phone making necessary calls to my mother and others that I knew would pray and support us through this latest bout of breast cancer. I tried not to be disappointed. Instead, encouragement came through the prayer support. I knew that it was the prayers of God's people that had sustained me in the past. I knew that I needed all the prayers I could receive this time as well.

At this time, we were between churches and did not yet have a church home. How different this round of cancer would be without our church family to comfort us. We were used to having a church family as a prayer and support team in the midst of our crises. Little did we know how many things would be different in comparing the two episodes of breast cancer. This was only the beginning.

All manner of thoughts began to plague my mind. The first one that came to me was that we had wasted a lot of money on a perfectly good breast reduction. But, no, I could not think that way. It was *through* the breast reduction that the cancer had been found. The second thought that came to my mind was that I *knew* that I should have had my breasts removed when I had the breast cancer the first time around. I was advised not to have this done because I was so young at the time. Yet I knew I had gone through the radiation treatments and all the discomforts for a reason, so I reminded myself not to play the game of what ifs.

The third thought that came to my mind was that I was not supposed to have breast cancer again! I had nearly a one hundred percent chance of never experiencing cancer again after the first time. Why did I have to experience this all over again? What didn't I learn the first time around? How much more will I have to go through? I wanted to enjoy life. I wanted to be carefree and happy.

June helped me initially with my inner turmoil. The Lord had provided June to be with me at this time. Her stepdaughter had experienced breast cancer at a young age. June had common sense, as well as a knowledge of the emotions I was experiencing and a heart sensitive to the Lord. The Lord has always been faithful to me in placing individuals in my life at selective moments to assist me on this path of life that God has for me.

My joy of a new life with a reduced bust had vanished. Feelings of disappointment, sorrow, fear, and anger replaced the newfound freedom of smaller breasts.

Hearing the news of cancer once again, I turned inward. I did not want to talk with people in person or over the telephone. I sent and received e-mails as well as cards through the mail, but that was the extent of it. I knew that people meant well, but even positive comments did not erase my negative state of mind. This was the time I wanted to have only my husband and daughters surrounding me. The giving and receiving of love was plentiful in our household. Love had always sustained us through traumatic times.

In a few days, I met with my oncologist. He gave me the news that I expected. I had done all the prescribed things to battle the breast cancer. I had endured the six and a half weeks of radiation treatments. I had taken the prescription of Tamoxifen. These were tools to prevent having cancer again. In my body, these tools had not worked. My only chance for survival now was a bilateral mastectomy. I needed all breast tissue removed. I was okay with this decision, and I was thankful I did not need to go through any form of chemotherapy. My oncologist assured me that was not necessary. Fortunately, once again the breast cancer had been discovered in its early stages. I was very grateful for this news.

The next step was to schedule an appointment with my surgeon. He was becoming way too familiar with my anatomy in my estimation! His kindness and concern for me were reassuring. He asked me when I wanted to have my double mastectomy done. My only response was to get it done as quickly as possible. If I had any more cancer lurking in my breast tissue, I wanted it out of there.

Examining the incisions from the breast reduction surgery, my surgeon readily agreed he could use the same incisions to perform the mastectomy. A simple bilateral mastectomy meant only breast tissue would be removed. The muscles and lymph nodes would be kept in place. Of course, I only had lymph nodes on the right side. Again, I was grateful for this bit of news.

We decided October 20, 2003, was the day for the double mastectomy. This gave me twenty days of having the perfect-sized breasts! Ken and I had to joke about this. What else could we do?

There was a word of caution from my surgeon. He explained to me I would have a more difficult time bouncing back with two surgeries less than three weeks apart. My thinking was that if I must again recuperate from surgery, I wanted to get it all over with at once. It made sense to Ken and me.

The twenty days in between surgeries seemed more like twenty years. At last, the day came for the double mastectomy. I knew that the Lord would be with me through this surgery as He had in the past. I drew on strength from the prayers of God's people and knowing that God was in control of the present, as well as the past and future.

I woke up in the recovery room of the hospital only to find I was in extreme discomfort. The pain was excruciating from the neck to the waistline, covering the front and sides of my torso. It was the worst pain I had felt in all of the surgeries combined together. It was as if I was on fire with pain. I immediately asked the nurse for assistance in pain medication.

The gurney ride to my hospital room was most unpleasant. Every bump, large or small, was felt in my midsection. What happened to me in the operating room? Why was I in so much pain? I didn't have that much breast tissue left to remove. It did not make sense to me. The attending nurse in my hospital room put her stethoscope to my chest and I thought of a boulder squashing an ant. I yelled out in sheer pain, and my nurse seemed surprised at my discomfort. It was one of those "duh" moments. I just had my breasts removed, why wouldn't it hurt? My yelling out got the nurse's attention and she backed off, attempting to be gentler with her approach to what was left of my body.

Huge bandages covered the area where my breasts had been. Four draining tubes were attached, two on the front and two on the sides. My mobility was limited because of these draining tubes. A very long needle was attached to each drain tube. When I would bend of any degree or even move, it felt like a needle jabbing me, which was actually the case. I was alive but feeling very hollow, inside and out.

CHAPTER ELEVEN

You have said, "I am overwhelmed with trouble!
Haven't I had enough pain already? And now the
Lord has added more! I am worn out from sighing
and can find no rest."

Jeremiah 45:3

Upon receiving my permission, a staff nurse at the hospital visited me. She had experienced a double mastectomy twelve years before. She was a ray of sunshine to me. She brought me little breast cancer survival gifts, like a breast cancer pin, a refrigerator magnet that said, "What Cancer Cannot Do," other little trinkets, and a brochure on the subject of breast cancer, which were all in a breast cancer tote bag. Her visits with me while I was in the hospital brought strength and encouragement to me.

At my first opportunity, I asked her why I was experiencing so much pain from this surgery. She explained that the surgeon, upon opening me up, had to use his fingers and *peel the breast tissue* out, much like peeling an orange. Breast tissue covers a vast area, not just the specific breast, thus the overwhelming pain and discomfort.

This explanation did not take away the pain, but it helped me to better deal with it and what was going on in my body. I did not recognize my body. I did not have enough time to adjust to my new body after the breast reduction. I was still in shock at the enormous change in my physical appearance. After all, for thirty-four years I had grown accustomed to having protruding breasts. Granted, they had grown considerably after having children. I had marks on my midsection from where my breasts had sagged against my torso all those years. Later calculations proved that a total of eight pounds of breast tissue had been removed by the two surgeries.

I welcomed visitors while I was in the hospital. Everyone wanted to hug me, and I wanted to hug everyone. It was next to impossible with the pain in my upper chest. We learned to hug with the head only. Anything touching the neck to the waist hurt me immensely.

Linda came to visit me. She herself was scheduled for open-heart surgery on that Friday of the same week. We could not get over the irony of the two of us having serious surgeries so closely together! We would later be recuperating at our own homes for several weeks, longing for the day we could get out and have lunch together again.

My sister Pat and her husband, Lee, came to visit me. They seemed to be in shock, as most people were, at the sight of my radically changed appearance. Not enough people had seen me after the breast reduction to know that change and now this even more drastic change. Everyone, myself included, was happy that the cancer had been removed once again and that the prognosis was good.

In fact, the second day in the hospital I received the pathology report, stating that there was no more cancer found in the excised breast tissue when the double mastectomy was performed. My initial reaction was a hallelujah celebration in the hospital bed. I called Ken at work to let him know the news he so urgently needed to hear. There were others I had to call immediately to let them know the good news.

The Lord was so good to me! After all, cancer had been eradicated. Once again, it was found to be true that early detection is the best protection. I would be free to go on living my life, altered as it were, but yet somehow I would be made whole again even with pieces and parts missing.

I was approached by my surgeon and others about having reconstructive surgery with implants. The thought of another surgery was the last thing on my mind. I was aware that some women chose that route, but I was mesmerized by being caved in and flat chested. In time, perhaps I would get some breast prostheses or forms to wear, but for now, I needed to heal and adjust to the new body I had.

I also had some female family members who did not encourage me to have implants, as the safety of them was still in question. For me, personally, I knew that I was not to have the implants. I knew if I had the implants, I would go on with life, forgetting the breast cancer had ever happened and living life to the max once again. I knew the Lord wanted me to be marked as a breast cancer survivor to be able to help other women. For me, that meant the daily reminder of God's goodness to my life and the lives of my husband and two daughters. Our daughters were now old enough to remember Mommy's breast cancer. They would remember Mommy with big boobies and Mommy with no boobies. Most importantly, they wanted their mommy around for keeps.

Unfortunately, I entertained thoughts of regret for having the double mastectomy performed. Earlier I had been exhilarated with the news, and then I found myself entertaining thoughts of how unnecessary this surgery had been since no more cancer had been found from the double mastectomy surgery. I could have had my perfect-sized breasts for life! Tears began to fill my eyes. I could not dwell on this. I had to tell myself that it was not a waste, that it was necessary to take all my breast tissue so there would not be any future occurrences of breast cancer. I was alive, and I needed to celebrate life every day that the Lord saw fit to give me life and breath.

I was able to go home by Wednesday evening after spending two nights in the hospital. Surely, I was strong enough to go home. On the short ride across town, I felt every inch of uneven road surface in my midsection. Even though it was good to be home, it was difficult. Getting comfortable in any position was next to impossible.

My parents were staying in our home, taking care of the girls' needs. They asked if I wanted them to stay longer now that I was home. I knew I needed help, and I gladly welcomed them staying a few more days.

I was allowed to sponge-bathe, but I found I did not have the strength nor could I maneuver with the four drain tubes. It was a humbling experience to ask my seventy-five-year-old mother to help bathe me, a grown woman of forty-four! She knew it was difficult for me to even ask her for help. She remembered I was her one child who always said to her, "I can do it myself!"

It was precarious wearing clothes of any kind. I had my four drain tubes that had to be pinned to my clothing. I attempted to conceal them, to hide the draining of blood they contained. I had trouble wearing anything, even elastic, around my waist, as I was still swollen and tender from the peeling of breast tissue that extended over my midsection. The other problem was my shirts hung on me. This was a good problem to have! My friend June had lost weight and graciously gave me some of her shirts that no longer fit her but fit me perfectly! This was indeed a blessing and something I had not thought about in the process of dealing with breast cancer again.

On Thursday, I welcomed my first guests into our home. Actually, Ed and Judy Aubuchon, my friends and now former senior pastor, needed a place to hang out while their house was being shown, hopeful that it would sell quickly. Judy, upon seeing me, replied, "Why, Karen, you look so cute. You look like a teeny-bopper with your flat chest!" In time, as I was exposed to other friends, it was the consensus that my double mastectomy had taken years off my physical appearance. This baby boomer was thrilled about that younger looking appearance for sure!

On Friday, I was scheduled to return to my surgeon to have my four drain tubes removed. My parents and Mackenzie accompanied me. I learned to ride in the car with a pillow on my front to protect my caved-in chest from the shoulder seatbelt. Unfortunately, I was disappointed to learn that only two of the drain tubes could be removed. They were giving me so much discomfort. I was still draining too much blood from the outer two tubes, so those had to remain for a few more days.

The surgeon also removed the bandage over my incisions. This was very traumatic to me. I hurt and I cried. My mother, filled with compassion, hurt with me. This was difficult on my parents to watch their daughter go through so much pain and discomfort. But they knew I was strong and that my faith was even stronger.

We picked up Allison from school and went home. With Ken home for the weekend, we decided my parents could return home that afternoon. They had been gone from their home from Sunday evening through Friday afternoon. This was a long time for these retired farmers to be gone from home.

The following Monday, I returned to the surgeon to finally get the other two drain tubes removed. What a relief that was! I was free of the apparatus attached to me.

Initially, after the surgery in the days and weeks that followed, I was fascinated by my new body. Looking at myself didn't bother me. I looked at myself from a scientific perspective as well as being so grateful to the Lord for my life spared! God was so good to me!

I was fortunate to have a husband who loved me consistently no matter if I had breasts or not. Ken liked the new look I now possessed. I was enjoying being flat chested for the first time in thirty-four years!

There were adjustments to make. Holding or carrying something under my arm was different, as the breast no longer held it in place. A few times, I found items dropping to the floor, as I was not proportioned for keeping them stable under my arm anymore.

One of the biggest adjustments was sleeping. I spent weeks once again sleeping in the recliner, as it was too painful to lie in bed. When I was finally able to try sleeping in bed, I clutched a pillow to replace the cushion provided by my breasts while sleeping on my side. Later, as I weaned myself from a pillow, I had to relearn comfortable positions for my arms to rest without breasts. It took time to learn new habits.

Confident that I was mending well and would soon be back to normal again, I started sending out résumés and making phone call interviews. It was all a facade. I did not sense the Lord's guiding hand for me to be a worship pastor again even as I pursued employment in this capacity. I knew it was what people expected of me. I knew deep down the Lord had other plans for my ministry.

By November 1, Ken and I believed it was time to put our home on the market. We believed that the Lord would be moving us on soon. At least that's what we told ourselves. We could not see the future living in our current home since our burden and calling for the church and community was all in the past.

I began to experience an emotional roller coaster ride that I was not prepared for. My oncologist had taken me off Tamoxifen. I had no idea what ramifications that, along with the removal of hormones with the double mastectomy, would have on my body. I was constantly irritable. I had hot flashes and night sweats that would almost take me beyond endurance. I became Ken's furnace in our bed. Winter was approaching, but in bed, it was in the heat of summer.

I did not want to be around people. I did not know if people would or could accept me now. I had become an alien. I was a minister of God's Word and loved being around people, but that was lost now. Survival was the key. I became content to sit in my recliner and observe the world through my laptop computer. I did not want to leave the house. I felt so conspicuous with my flat chest. I had thoughts of wearing a sign across my chest that read, "Yes, I had breast cancer again, and my breasts are gone!"

This was foreign territory to me. I was not accustomed to sitting in a corner and licking my wounds. In the past, I had always been a social butterfly and wanted people around me. Now I only wanted to isolate myself from people. I was all alone. No one could help me. Could I survive change in my body mentally and emotionally?

Doors of ministry opportunities would open and close right before my eyes. Inwardly, I did not feel strong enough to handle another ministerial position. I had been beat down in my physical body, and it was affecting my spiritual self as well. I began to question if I even knew the will of God or what He wanted from me.

The winter months brought a depression that settled into the very depths of my being. Thoughts of God abandoning me were constant. Every direction I turned, it seemed as though God had abandoned me. I held on to God's Word because I knew this was a lie from the devil. God had not abandoned me, no matter what had happened to me. I clung to Hebrews 13:5: "For God has said, 'I will never fail you. I will never abandon you.'"

A glimmer of hope would start to surface in my mind. But it always seemed to be short lived. It was as if God had left me on a deserted island to fend for myself. Where was God when I needed Him the most? No matter how much I cried out to Him, all was silent. I still questioned God and His plan for my life. What was He thinking? What was He doing with me?

Blood tests were run in January during my six-month checkup with my oncologist. The blood work revealed my liver levels were elevated. This got the attention of my oncologist. He was not sure the reason for this and wanted me to make a return visit in two weeks to evaluate these levels. Fortunately, later blood work returned the liver levels back to near normal. It was discovered the cause for the elevated levels was a result of going off Tamoxifen at the time of my bilateral mastectomy.

By the end of February, I was ready to be fitted for breast forms. I had no idea what to expect or what to choose. I had the choice of perky breasts but realized that did not look natural. I knew I wanted small breasts. Choosing a size six breast form was my new look! It was similar to my size after the breast reduction.

Breast-form bras were part of the package. There again, I had no idea what I wanted or needed. It took months of wearing the breast forms and bras before I learned what did and did not work for me.

I was thankful for good health insurance that paid for most of the cost of the breast forms and bras. I realized I was still making adjustments to a new body and a new look. My natural inhibitions made me feel self-conscious. I was sure that everybody was looking at my caved-in chest, knowing good and well how large I had previously been.

My caved-in chest made me recall a childhood memory. I enjoyed playing with Barbie dolls as a child. Barbie and Ken's friends, Midge and Alan, were the first two dolls I had in that collection. Using my imagination one day, I used a desk lamp to pretend Alan was sunbathing. Before long, I realized his chest had caved in from the heat of the desk lamp. Thoughts of my chest looking like my doll Alan gave me a good laugh.

March 1, 2004, was the official launch date of the ministry I believed God had birthed in me years earlier. It would be called *Path of Life Ministries*. It was based on the Scripture He had given me originally at the beginning of the breast cancer in 2000: "You have made known to me the path of life; you will fill me with joy in your presence, with eternal pleasures at your right hand" (Psalm 16:11, NIV).

Finding joy in His presence seemed to be unattainable because of everything I had negatively experienced. Oh, how I longed for that joy. Was it possible?

CHAPTER TWELVE

A prayer of one overwhelmed with trouble, pouring out problems before the Lord. Lord, hear my prayer! Listen to my plea!

Psalm 102:1

Outwardly, I appeared to be adjusting well to my new, altered body. Inwardly, I struggled with life, wondering if I would ever experience any normalcy again. I doubted myself in so many ways. How did I appear to people? Those who did not know me did not know anything was different. Those who did know me knew I had undergone a tremendous body change.

If asked, I would have denied feeling like an animal going into hiding to lick its wounds. In reality, that is exactly what I had done. I knew I desperately needed a support group but could not bring myself to it. I feared that if I leaned upon a support group, I would unravel and the tears would flow in torrents. I had two daughters watching me and my every move. I must remain strong.

Allison and Mackenzie had questions. First of all, they wondered if their mommy was going to die. They mistakenly thought the words *surgery* and *cancer* were synonymous. Ken and I would take the time to explain various aspects of my situation to the girls. We wanted the girls to accept reality and learn how to handle the tough times in life.

Financially, we struggled. Refinancing our house a second time during the course of less than two years brought some relief. Too many surgeries too close together were an added financial strain that made it difficult to make ends meet. It was as if I was put out to pasture in the ministry. I no longer brought any income to the family. I toyed with the feeling of vindication. After all, I had worked and provided for the family totally while Ken was unemployed a few years earlier. I had done my part. Those thoughts quickly dissipated out of love for my husband and daughters.

My motives for working were not entirely selfless, however. If I could work full-time, I would not have to face my own demons. I could get on with life. I could keep so busy I would not have to think about breast cancer again. Perhaps I could better accept these physical changes if I was working full time.

My new ministry, *Path of Life Ministries,* was off to a slow start. I still had the vision, but I didn't know how to get from point A to point B. I needed an instruction manual on how to get a ministry going.

I struggled with my breast forms. I did not enjoy wearing them full time. I wanted to feel free and go without them. I did not want to look weird, though, out in public. Ken referred to my breast forms as a convertible, since I could go with or without them. I was learning the appropriateness of the breast forms. My college-aged niece and a guy friend of hers came to assist Ken and me with some yard work. Thinking it was appropriate to wear the breast forms because of this strange young man in our home, I wore them. As we finished dinner and proceeded to the backyard to work, the work was quite physical. With sweat and movement, I discovered my breast forms were creeping toward my neck! I quickly excused myself to the house where I removed the breast forms. I discreetly explained to my niece what had happened. She thought it was hysterically funny, as did I. We did not tell the guys.

By early summer of 2004, I had developed what looked to be a pimple. It did not heal after a few days. I soon realized it was a boil, not a pimple. After messing with it for a month, I finally saw my doctor. She recommended an antibiotic to see if that would heal it. Two weeks later, I was not any better. I began to be concerned about this boil not healing, as I wondered if it was cancerous. After being through cancer of any kind, it changes a person to notice any little thing in or on the body. The first question in the mind is always, "Is it cancer?"

As I went back to my doctor, she recommended lancing the boil. An appointment was set with my surgeon. This was a simple, outpatient procedure to lance the boil. My surgeon referred to it as a cyst. Thankfully, it was taken care of rapidly. The difficult part came in waiting for the pathology report. A few days later, I received the call from my surgeon's office, stating that the surgically removed cyst revealed no cancer. Ken and I were very relieved to hear this news.

Menopausal symptoms played havoc with my emotional, mental, and physical well-being. The minute I thought I had one symptom under control, another reared its ugly head. There were times I thought I was losing my mind. I thought about pioneer women and how they suffered and endured this momentous time in their lives. Every woman had to deal with this time of life. The alternative was death, and death was not an option for me. I knew that God wanted me to live, He had a purpose and a plan for my life, and I had a husband and two daughters who needed me. I wanted to live, so I knew I had to overcome these obstacles. I could do this no other way but with the Lord's help and strength.

I had begun to receive some ministry opportunities to speak at some churches in which we introduced and promoted Path of Life Ministries. This was very exciting for me! I definitely knew this was what the Lord wanted me to do. This was what I was anointed to do! I preached with passion and fervor, wanting to help others find their path of life.

Even though positive things were happening, the darkness continued to lurk deep inside of me. Could I ever truly accept the outward changes to my body? What made me a woman? Are breasts what define a woman? There was only so much encouragement Ken could give me. He loved me unconditionally. He loved me consistently. He was most patient with me.

I found myself renting movies such as *Elephant Man*, *The Man Without a Face*, and *Phantom of the Opera* in hopes of finding some understanding. These were movies in which individuals had to learn to live with their own deformities. Could I live with myself now? These movies did not bring the answers for which I longed. Watching movies was an outlet of escaping the world in which I now lived. I could not go back. I would never have my breasts again. It was a huge bodily loss, not only emotionally, but physically as well. A part of me wanted to believe God for the ultimate miracle. After all, God can do anything. He could "grow" breasts, beautiful breasts on my body to replace the concave chest. Why should God do this? Was it my own vanity? Were my breasts what made me a woman? Did my breasts define who I was?

Before I knew it, fall was here. School started. I had been warned about this event and the emotional impact it would have on me. My baby daughter started kindergarten! Thankfully, Mackenzie went on Mondays, Wednesdays, and Fridays. I still had her on Tuesdays and Thursdays. Initially, this new chapter of my life and Mackenzie's was not a drastic adjustment.

Ken and I were not surprised to learn that Mackenzie was the oldest student in her kindergarten class. She had missed the cutoff date by nine days to begin kindergarten the year before. It was difficult the year before, as Mackenzie was extremely ready to begin kindergarten. I had questioned why this had to be. The law is the law. It was then, however, that I recognized God's plan for my own personal needs. I cherished having Mackenzie at home with me while I was recuperating from the bilateral mastectomy. Her little presence gave me the knowledge that life was not all about me. I needed to give and receive love from Mackenzie.

She provided a healing balm during those critical first days and weeks of my recovery.

I could understand now why so many women wanted to have another baby when their last child left for kindergarten. In our case, this was physically impossible. We were happy with the two daughters we knew the Lord had blessed us with.

The restlessness inside me continued to grow. I now had time on my hands. With both girls attending the Christian school, finances were stretched to the max. I was not contributing very much financially with my preaching opportunities. This put a tremendous burden on my shoulders to do my part for the sake of our family's welfare. Ken never put this burden on me; it was self-inflicted. He just wanted me happy and healthy.

I learned of a pastoral care minister opening at the church we were attending. This appealed to me, so I applied for the position. I even had an interview. But, deep in my heart, I knew this was not the Lord's direction. Why was I pursuing it then? I even pursued opportunities online, attempting to make some extra income by filling out surveys. This became a pastime and was taking up a good deal of my time. Was this what the Lord had in mind for me? Would I be able to help with some of the financial load? I was hopeful. Day after day, week after week, month after month went by before I realized things are not always as they appear. I made very little income.

I saw an ad for a childcare environment where I could work part-time as a teacher. I began to pursue this possibility. It was a positive learning environment for children with pleasant personnel. *I could do this,* I determined.

What I had failed to do was ask the Lord if this was what He wanted me to do. There are times in our lives that we get in a mess because we have done our own thing. Then, almost as an afterthought, we think to ask God's blessings on our endeavors. And then it comes as a surprise when the Lord speaks to our hearts, telling us this was not His idea in the first place. God still had a better plan. The part-time employment this job offered was afternoon and early evenings. I soon learned this would not work with our family schedule. Ken has learned over the years to let me make my own decisions, even though I ask him for his blessing. We halfway closed the door on this job opportunity, as I volunteered to continue as a substitute when necessary.

It was a bittersweet time. Often, I felt like screaming. I wanted God to get me out of this rut my life had become. I still felt like He had put me on a shelf, and I wondered if He would ever get me down again and use me for His kingdom. It seemed like every door of opportunity I opened, the Lord soundly closed in my face. But after all, isn't this what we pray for the Lord to do if it is not His will? Still, I was frustrated with God, with life, and with people in general. Had I truly accepted myself and this new outward appearance? On the surface, I thought I had. No one knew how I still did battle on the inside and how I longed for the emotional healing that I still so desperately needed. The physical healing of my scars was obvious; the emotional scarring was much slower to heal.

CHAPTER THIRTEEN

Though we are overwhelmed by our sins, you
forgive them all.

Psalm 65:3

I threw myself into biblical study and online
research. This led me to a Web site for retreats. Part of
my vision for Path of Life Ministries was speaking at
retreats in a small group setting where women could
feel free to share openly. I listed Path of Life Ministries
on this Web site, hoping to get some insight on this
endeavor. I had no idea what I was doing, but there
was an excitement stirring inside me. This was a good
sign, I knew.

One evening I took a call from a lady interested in
one of my retreats. This was news to me! I thought I
was just the speaker, not the organizer of the retreat. It
was through this phone call the Lord spoke gently to
my heart and helped me to envision what I must do.

I secured a retreat house at a local conference center
campground with the thought, *If I build it, they will*

come. I had had doubts about our location being an ideal setting for what we had in mind. With those doubts, the Lord assured me there were needs all around; it did not matter where we held the retreat. He would be there meeting the needs of those who came. I was only the facilitator; the Holy Spirit was the One totally responsible for the outcome. The same day I booked the retreat house, I received a letter of acknowledgment stating I had not been chosen for the pastoral care minister position. Instead of being disappointed, I was elated, knowing this time I was in the center of God's will. It had been a long time since I had sensed the Lord's divine direction in our lives.

The next thing I knew, I received a telephone call from one of the presbyters in the state, asking me if I could preach at a church that was without a pastor. The phone call came on a Friday afternoon, and it was for that Sunday morning and evening services. Instead of panic, I exclaimed enthusiastically I would be happy to fill in! Getting asked to preach at a church was like receiving a shot of vitamins. I already had a message stirring in my heart, so I was well on my way. The remainder of 2004 took us to this church four weekends to minister in both the morning and evening services. Our daughters became fast friends with the other children at this church. Ken and I had an excitement stirring in us for this congregation. They were a warm group of people who were easy to love.

Our vacation was set for Christmas break from the school. Exploring the southwest part of the United States made for a wonderful vacation, putting over 3,000 miles on our Grand Cherokee Jeep. Our family loves adventure and travel, which was exactly what we had planned for this vacation.

Two days before we left on vacation, I noticed a pain under my rib cage on the right side. I did not want anything to change our vacation plans, which included spending Christmas with one of Ken's brothers and his parents. I decided to watch what I ate and not eat much, hoping that would help. I managed well under this regimen.

Upon returning home right after the New Year of 2005, I noticed the pain once again. Day after day, I fought with the pain. It was a nagging pain, though usually not intense. I tried ignoring it, thinking it would go away.

The childcare employment was reopened with a different opportunity. This time it was teaching music to three and four-year-olds. It had a complete program to follow. Surely, I could do this; it was right up my alley. I began to prepare for it. Right away, I noticed it was more physical than musical, which was not my usual approach to teaching music. After all, I had to consider the audience! That age needed to be physical in order to learn the basics. What had I gotten myself into?

Mackenzie became very sick. Struggling with a fever for three days, I took her to the pediatrician on the same day I had my six-month checkup with my oncologist. Mackenzie had an eye and ear infection. She was put on an antibiotic and given drops for her eyes.

I had been so focused on Mackenzie and getting her well that I had put my own pain aside. I told my oncologist about the pain and other abnormalities I was noticing. The look of concern on his face said it all. He scheduled a CAT scan for the next day. We had to rule out cancer, first and foremost. I did not even want to think that way but knew this was a precautionary procedure.

Even though I knew the CAT scan was routine, my mind still wandered to the what ifs. I had to convince myself I would be fine; I had so much to do. In the meantime, I vacillated between bouts of nausea and diarrhea.

That Thursday morning after the CAT scan, Ken and I drove to the retreat house so he could envision the environment we would be working in. I was thankful Ken had taken the day off to be with me and to watch Mackenzie since she wasn't in school that day.

Plenty was on my mind. I was asked to lead the praise and worship as well as preach that Sunday morning at a church in the area. I was heavily into planning and organizing for this retreat now scheduled for February 4 through 6. With seven sessions of teaching slated for this retreat, there was much studying and research to accomplish. I also had the teaching position for the childcare employment that was to begin on Friday.

Friday morning came. I expected to hear from my oncologist for the results of the CAT scan. In the meantime, I got myself ready to go teach the little three- and four-year-olds.

Just as I was walking out the door, the telephone rang. It was my oncologist. He said he did not have good news. It appeared there were spots on my liver that were cancerous. He wanted to schedule a liver biopsy for Tuesday of the following week.

I got off the telephone in near hysteria. All I could say was, "No, no, no! I will not have cancer again! No!" I was not in a frame of mind to teach small children, so I called the director to tell her what had just transpired. She needed the teaching material, so I told her I would drop it off to her shortly. I knew then I could not do the job of music instruction for the children. I realized I had taken on too much, and now another cancer scare had raised its ugly head. The specter of another round of cancer was almost more than I could bear. As I headed out the door to drop off tennis shoes for one of the girls at school, I attempted to stifle tears, but nevertheless they flowed like a spring rain. In a state of numbness, I ran by the childcare employment to drop off the music materials. The director was very concerned about my health. I drove on endlessly around town, attempting to call Ken over and over. I could not get him by phone. The irony was that he worked for a telephone company. He not only had an office phone, but two cell phones. I tried all three phones for thirty minutes before I finally reached him. By this time, I had found myself at Linda's house once again. I had earlier joked with her that I would be fine unless she found me on her doorstep.

Here I was—at Linda's doorstep—my haven of refuge away from home. She, too, was in a state of shock once I shared the news from my oncologist. We sat in silence. I felt no peace. Where was the peace of God in all of this?

Sharing the news with Ken was difficult. His voice revealed his love and concern for me. He asked me not to be alone, but to stay at Linda's house if possible. He would come as soon as he could get away. Linda asked if I would like for her to call her pastor and I agreed. He arrived in just a matter of minutes. The three of us sat, talked, drank coffee, and tried to sort all of this out. Questions of *why is this happening again* hung in the air like a vapor.

I thought my life would soon be over if this was liver cancer. I had watched others with liver cancer and knew that with that diagnosis came a short life expectancy. I did not want this. I knew God had a purpose and plan for my life, and heaven was not on the agenda, at least not yet. We had daughters to raise who needed both a mother and a father. Anyone who tells you that hearing the diagnosis of cancer over and over again becomes easier or commonplace simply is being untruthful. I felt numb. It was as though time stood still. How many times must I walk this path, feel this dread, suffer this terror?

Ken arrived at Linda's house. We embraced for a long time. He told me he made arrangements for the girls to spend the night at my sister and brother-in-law's house thirty miles away. We needed time alone to sort this out in our own minds before sharing it with our daughters and other family members.

Linda's pastor prayed a genuine and lengthy prayer regarding this latest development. Through his prayer, I began to feel God's peace. God would see me through this, whatever it involved. He had always remained faithful. Why would this time be any different?

I held on to Psalm 118:17: "I will not die; instead, I will live to tell what the Lord has done." This was the verse my mother had held onto when she went through her bout of cancer, and now I would make it mine. I determined to live.

CHAPTER FOURTEEN

We think you ought to know, dear brothers and
sisters, about the trouble we went through ... We
were crushed and overwhelmed beyond our
ability to endure, and we thought we would
never live through it.

2 Corinthians 1:8

Ken and I chose not to immediately share this
news of possible cancer with our families until it was
absolutely necessary. We did confide in Lee and Pat
since they had graciously kept our daughters overnight.
We believed it only fair to tell them. Upon sharing our
news, Lee asked me if he could pray for me. I agreed
readily. I knew that Lee had a way about him. He could
powerfully touch the throne of God when he prayed
for a person. This time would prove to be no exception.

We also told Allison and Mackenzie what was going
on. They had many questions, and we answered them
as well as we could.

I contacted the e-mail prayer chain of our Assemblies of God district's ministers. Shortly after that e-mail hit everyone's computers, I instantly felt strengthened with the prayers of God's people. Phone calls were received from fellow ministers who wanted to pray with me over the telephone. I was in no position to turn away any prayers, and all were welcomed. I knew God would hear and answer the prayers of His people. We still chose to wait as far as telling our families the news. I could not bear to give my mother any more cancer-related news about me.

Tuesday, the day of the liver biopsies, came finally. It had seemed like a long weekend with the results of the CAT scan coming in on Friday morning. Ken took off work to be with me. The girls were in school. We had arranged for Linda to pick them up from school and keep them until we got home from the hospital.

I was petrified of this procedure. There were many steps to go through before the actual biopsies took place. The last step involved my instructions during the biopsies. I would lie on my stomach while the needle and scope would be inserted in my back where the liver was located. I was told most people were fearful of this procedure, but after it was finished, decided it wasn't really that bad. I only wished I could believe this was true. I could not be sedated enough. I had to remain awake and alert in order to follow the breathing instructions, which were to breathe in, breathe out, hold. This occurred over and over for approximately thirty minutes. My arms had to be over my head. I clutched the pillow that lay under my head. Tears flowed from time to time with the intense pain of the needle in my liver. It felt as if a dagger had been inserted and then twisted, over and over again. Two biopsies of the liver were performed.

I was supposed to be in the recovery room for four hours. Because of my blood pressure nearly bottoming out and the loss of blood, there was some concern. I was finally dismissed from the hospital at six thirty that evening, hours later than originally planned.

Ken took me home first before picking up the girls at Henry and Linda's house. The girls greeted me with somber and grave looks on their little faces. I tried reassuring them I would be fine, but that I was very sore and weak from the procedure I had undergone. Still, I could sense Allison was doing her best to be a brave little girl. As she began talking to me, her lower lip quivered, and I knew she was fighting back tears. In pain or not, I grabbed hold of Allison and Mackenzie, holding them and loving them for a long time. My sweet babies had seen their mother go through so much pain and suffering in their short lives.

Once again, the misconception the girls had was that surgery and cancer were synonymous. Ken and I talked to them, pointing out that was not necessarily the case.

For the next two days, I found myself weak from the procedure. My mind replayed over and over the needle twisting in my back. I remained uncomfortable.

By the second day, the results were confirmed. One liver biopsy revealed a benign tumor on my liver. The other biopsy of the liver was still in question.

An MRI was the next step to determine what was wrong with me. Again, Tuesday was the scheduled day for the MRI. Linda was able to go with me this time so Ken would not have to take off work. I needed somebody to be with Mackenzie while I had the MRI.

When I went into that *tube,* instantly Psalm 91:1 came to my mind: "Those who live in the shelter of the Most High will find rest in the shadow of the Almighty." The Lord was blanketing me with His love and care in the midst of the enclosure of the MRI. I found myself using this opportunity to pray. I let my imagination wonder over the various noises in the MRI. Again, I was given the instructions to breathe in, breathe out, breathe in again, and hold. I rejoiced that the MRI was not painful, unlike the liver biopsies.

By four thirty that same afternoon, I received a telephone call from my oncologist with the emphatic and triumphant news of no cancer! I did a hallelujah dance all over the house. I had not expected to hear so soon from my oncologist, which made this good news even sweeter.

On one hand, I was still rejoicing, but on the other hand, the pain lingered. My oncologist referred me to my primary physician. Upon telling her my symptoms, she believed it was a bad gallbladder. She ordered the hydro-scan, the ultimate test to diagnose a bad gallbladder.

I had already been put through the mill, so one more test was only routine for me. Once again, this test was scheduled for the next Tuesday. It seemed my tests were *always* on Tuesdays. This was a habit that I wanted to see broken rapidly!

The hydro-scan test was smooth sailing. It was the easiest test I had endured. Lying perfectly still for thirty minutes while being scanned nearly put me to sleep!

The results of the hydro-scan test proved that my gallbladder was bad. I met with my surgeon on Thursday. His schedule for surgeries was full for Friday morning, but upon my pleading, he scheduled me for first thing at 6:45 a.m. I always preferred early morning surgeries, as it gave me less time to think about what was happening.

My surgeon and I made a pact that this was the last surgery I would need. He told me enough was enough, and I more than agreed with him. Thankfully, this surgery was to be performed laparoscopically.

I called my parents to come and help out with the girls, which they willingly agreed to do. I felt badly putting my parents through yet another surgery, but there was nothing I could do. I needed help.

With the surgery scheduled for Friday, February 4, I had to cancel the Path of Life retreat I had scheduled for that weekend. No one had signed up for it, so it was just a matter of contacting the retreat center and postponing until another weekend.

My Sundays were full, preaching at various churches around the state. In preaching, I never wanted the focus to be on "poor Karen" and what she was going through at the time. I only wanted to give God the glory through my life and praise Him for what He continued to do in and through me. With each hardship and surgery came an increased compassion for people hurting with physical maladies.

The surgery could not come soon enough. As I was being prepped for surgery, Ken was by my side, loving me and praying for me. Tears came easily to my eyes. The nurse saw my tears and reassured me that everything would be fine with the surgery. He did not understand the tears. I did not want to go through another surgery. I was worn out from the weeks of tests and the years of surgeries. I turned my thoughts to the Lord, knowing that He would sustain me once again.

I woke up in the recovery room with the immediate knowledge that my pain was gone. I recalled my hysterectomy and thinking how I woke up from that surgery with no pain. Now it was just a matter of recuperating and gaining back my strength.

The first few nights at home were spent in my recliner, as that was the only comfortable position I could sleep in. My devoted husband sacrificially slept on the floor in the family room close by me so that I would not be alone. As a result, I slept beautifully.

With the gallbladder gone, I found myself eating minimally. If I ate very much, I would be in pain or discomfort. This was a wonderful diet plan, just cut back on the eating! It was then I believed the Lord spoke to my heart, encouraging me to lose some excess weight so I would find myself in a healthier state of well-being. Over the next several months, the weight was reduced by approximately thirteen pounds and a size smaller in clothing. How exciting this was to me!

The Path of Life retreat was rescheduled for May 13 through 15. My studying and researching for the teaching sessions were beneficial to those who attended the retreat. It was a small group setting, but the impact of the retreat was positive. The comments affirmed that this was a successful retreat!

With the summer fast approaching, Ken and I purposed in our hearts that this would be an excellent time to pursue job opportunities for him outside of the area. An opportunity quickly came in June. As a family, we traveled the 460 miles one way for the job interview for which Ken was hopeful. It was close to Ken's parents' house, giving our daughters some quality time with the grandparents they did not get to see very often.

So sure this was God's will and purpose for our lives, I secured a real estate agent. A friend of ours drove two hours to go house hunting with the real estate agent and me while Ken had his job interview. After looking at several houses, Ken finally called me with the good news that he had landed the job. It was now fine for us to get serious about finding a house. But, in my spirit, something did not seem to be right. This had been way too easy. I was so ready to move that I thought this had to be God's will.

When we announced our news of relocating to Ken's parents, their initial lack of enthusiasm alarmed me. Our daughters stared at us in disbelief. Mackenzie was full of questions but reasonably excited. On the other hand, Allison was tearful and upset. She did not want to move and leave her friends. We tried explaining to her that life was full of changes and there would be friends everywhere the Lord took us. It was not that easy for Allison to accept, however.

The 460-mile drive back home was full of hashing and rehashing the job interview. Ken needed to vent, and I knew the importance of talking things out. This was a big move in our lives. We needed to be sure this was God's will and not our own.

Ken had not accepted the job offer, as he wanted forty-eight hours to think and pray about it first. After this time had passed, he called the guy back to accept the job. However, there was some confusion involved during the course of the conversation.

This sense of confusion did not go away for Ken and me. In fact, it affected my nerves so much that I broke out in shingles by July 1. Shingles were on the left side of my face. The worst spot was right under my eye. It was puffy and darkened and resembled a black eye. At times, it felt like creepy crawlers scurrying all over the left side of my face. What an experience!

Shingles is caused by the same virus that causes chickenpox. If you have had chickenpox (over ninety percent of adults have), the virus remains in your body and can cause shingles. The chickenpox virus stays inactive in certain nerves. Conditions that weaken the body's immune system, such as cancer, increase the chance that the virus will become active again, resulting in the painful disease known as shingles. Excessive stress also increases the chance for the onset of shingles.

Due to several red flags rising up, by July 11, Ken came to the conclusion this was not the job for him to take. The communiqué between Ken and the guy he had interviewed with was ended.

Ken did not have chickenpox as a child, so we took every precaution to ensure that he would not contract the virus. He and I were prescribed a week's supply of Valtrex. In the mean time, he began the adult series of chickenpox vaccinations. The side effects for Valtrex were aggressive behavior, which made for an interesting seven days around the Norton house! Ken would come home from work, thoroughly exhausted from restraining himself from verbally assaulting his co-workers. I, on the other hand, expressed myself more strongly than I should have to Ken and the girls.

The shingles gradually subsided. I had a pit in my face under my left eye where the biggest shingle had located itself. I was hopeful that in time it would heal and not leave a noticeable scar. I did not want to be vain about my appearance, but it was awful having shingles on my face! A general feeling of malaise plagued me on a daily basis for several weeks. I fought depression continually.

All my life I had always pushed myself to the max, never recognizing my boundaries or limitations until it was too late. With the shingles, for the first time in my life, I had a warning signal. The shingles were over, but the nerve endings could again become irritated if I allowed myself to get overwhelmed. I taught myself to make a conscious effort to change directions emotionally and mentally. This was necessary to do to cause the nerve endings to completely heal and return to normal. This was a major time of learning for me. I had always let life happen to me instead of making the conscious effort to take control. Now I was making progress toward a more healthy emotional life.

CHAPTER FIFTEEN

No, despite all these things, overwhelming victory is ours through Christ, who loved us.

Romans 8:37

Life was beginning to make sense to me. I was growing spiritually by leaps and bounds. The struggles and trials with my physical health had weighed me down considerably. Thinking there was no end to poor physical health brought depression. However, this was not the end of life on this earth.

The Lord graciously taught me that He is everything I need at any point in the day, no matter what I may go through in this life. All my life I had looked to people to meet my emotional needs. It always seemed that God had provided people for me to latch onto. Unfortunately, I was disappointed over and over by people. No one person could fill all my emotional needs. People are people. God gives us people to be a blessing but also requires us to be a blessing in return. It's just that simple. Our most gracious Father God can meet all the emotional needs of anyone—even a complex person such as myself.

During the two *silent* years in which I felt like the Lord had put me on a shelf and was giving me a spiritual timeout, He taught me the proper perspective I should have with people. This made for smoother relationships with everybody. The difficulty I had had with loving some people was replaced by Christ's compassion in me. I was able to love them as Jesus loves them. On the other hand, the people I loved the dearest were no longer placed on a pedestal. I knew that the only one I was to worship and adore was my heavenly Father. Everyone else came second place.

It was fun to be with myself now. I could not get over the changes that were occurring in me. There continues to be times of sheer amazement over how much the Lord has changed and is changing me for the better! Truly, I identified with the scripture in Zephaniah 3:17: "For the Lord your God is living among you. He is a mighty savior. He will take delight in you with gladness. With his love, he will calm all your fears. He will rejoice over you with joyful songs." God was overwhelming me by His presence! I began to understand how I needed the kiss of God in my life. I could be overwhelmed by the intimacy in my relationship with my heavenly Father. There were no limitations with Him. I could envision myself climbing onto my heavenly Father's lap and resting there quietly in His loving arms.

I had always believed strongly in having a close relationship with my Lord and Savior. It is one thing to believe it and even think you are living it. To practice it, though, is a lifelong learning process. I was on the journey, on the path, learning to practice the presence of the Lord with me at all times. I did not have to be overwhelmed by my circumstances. My circumstances had taken me on a negative and downward spiral. This had happened to me consistently throughout my life. Now I could be constantly overwhelmed by the Lord's presence in my daily life. The choice was up to me. It had always been up to me, and now I understood.

Going through the breast cancer for the second time had taken its toll on me. I had always been able to release my emotions through music. The underlying depression that came with the cancer had robbed me of this outlet. What a tremendous revelation it was to know this! I had been on antidepressants to help me deal with this new dimension of living without certain body parts. I had been on various antidepressants during these years, trying to find the one that was best suited for my needs. I finally weaned myself off the antidepressants during the fall of 2004. I used Ken as my barometer in case I started going off the deep end. He watched me, though, and over a period of time, discovered that I was doing fine without the antidepressants. He observed how the antidepressants had kept me on an even keel through everyday life. Without the antidepressants, I was able to experience the highs and lows that life entailed. It was more exciting for Ken and me to enjoy life together this way!

I had put music, for the most part, aside during the last two years. I had no song to sing. There was no song in my heart. That part of me seemed to lie dormant as if I was in a season of winter. It had been a long winter.

Whether it was singing or playing a keyboard, I worshiped the Lord and allowed the intensity of my inner being to break forth in sorrow or jubilation. This was how the Lord specifically spoke to my heart—through music. That was always His best channel through which to speak to me. I began to see the Lord stirring up the love of music in my heart and spirit once again. For those two years, I attended one worship service after another, but my singing was not from my innermost being. I would not allow myself to go into deeper realms of worship and intimacy with the Lord. *But it's different now.*

The winter season was finally over, and spring had blossomed. The music was back in my heart and life. Now I wanted to express my love and devotion to the Lord through music once again. Joy was in my heart to stay. There was a peace in knowing I was special to God. Philippians 4:7 was powerful to me: "Then you will experience God's peace, which exceeds anything we can understand. His peace will guard your hearts and minds as you live in Christ Jesus." I may not understand why I had to endure so much in so few years, but I now had His peace.

The other issue that had been resolved in my thinking was that I could once again trust God with my life. He had not failed me or disappointed me. When life goes a different direction than what we expect, we sometimes turn inward and think the only one we can trust is ourselves. After a season of healing, we find our hearts returning to our heavenly Father, who is always trustworthy, even when we may not recognize this fact in our lives.

Once again, in the fall of 2005, I was put through some tests because of pain in my right flank. This time I was confident God was on my side and that nothing was wrong with me. The enemy of my soul wanted to overwhelm me once again and convince me that I would get cancer again. My heavenly Father desired that I walk in His path, and I was not alone. He is there with me, walking ever so closely beside me.

The outcome of those tests proved that nothing was wrong with me. It was soon revealed to me that it was a muscular soreness that took care of itself in a matter of a few weeks by changing how I went about doing some physical work.

Life is a constant journey. It involves taking one step at a time, one foot in front of the other. There are times when we would like to quit. Those times are the most precious, as our heavenly Father has sent His Holy Spirit to walk beside us—just as a best friend would, only so much better.

Quite often, I reflect on childhood memories of walking the path in my dad's field on the farm he owned. The path had some curves, but I could always see the western sky and the setting of the sun. As long as I could see the sun, I felt safe. The same is true with life: though we may not know what the curves in life may bring, as long as we sense the openness and warmth of Jesus, the Son of God, we are safe in His hands.

My roots for walking this life as a Christian began as a child in the openness and freedom to play in the field—running, skipping, or walking on the path. My desire to be all that I could ever be for God, loving

Him with all my mind, heart, and strength grew daily as a child and continues throughout life.

Will I fight cancer again? Only the Lord knows. I refuse to live my life in the shadows of fear and worry. That thought of impending cancer passed through my mind nearly every day for two years. The Lord has helped me with those thoughts. Second Corinthians 10:3–5 says, "We are human, but we don't wage war as humans do. We use God's mighty weapons, not worldly weapons, to knock down the strongholds of human reasoning and to destroy false arguments. We destroy every proud obstacle that keeps people from knowing God. We capture their rebellious thoughts and teach them to obey Christ."

Yes, cancer changes your life, but it does not have to end your life. Cancer did not take away my relationship with my heavenly Father.

I am convinced the Lord will see a person through anything. He will give the appropriate strength needed for the specific time of testing and trial in one's life. At times, one may think life is dishing out more than one can possibly bear or endure. He is there, embracing you, holding you, cheering you on: "You can make it, my child; you can make it!"

EPILOGUE

It is now 2010, and I can now objectively deal with the past and what the Lord took me through in those years of cancer; I am nearly seven years of being cancer free.

In retrospect, I see that it was quite necessary for me to go through all the cancers and surgeries that I did to make me a compassionate lead pastor now for over three years. Every time I visit someone in the hospital, I have a keen sense of what is going on which helps me to minister more effectively to those who are in the hospital. So many people have hurts in their lives. We live in a period of time where many people deal with cancer.

As our family continues to enjoy vacations where we go four-wheeling, the Lord often reminds me that the paths we are on are rocky, much like our very lives, but that He will go with us every inch of the way. There are times we cannot determine what is ahead. As we meet other vehicles who have already made the journey, it is proof to me that we, too, can make it. Just as Ken drives our Jeep over the rocks and I have no control except to pray and hang on to the handle, the Lord reminds me to trust Him as the driver and let Him maneuver over the rocky path that is ahead.

My desire is that this book will strengthen, encourage, and help those who are battling cancer, whether personally or someone close to you. Celebrate life—every single day of it—for as long as the Lord allows you on this earth! That is what I continue to do, my friend!

REFERENCES

1. Helen Reddy, Ray Burton. "I Am Woman." Buggerlugs Music, 1972.

2. John Ezzy, Daniel Grul, Steve McPherson. "Jesus Lover of My Soul." Hillsong, 1992.

CPSIA information can be obtained at www.ICGtesting.com
Printed in the USA
LVOW10s1733270116

472517LV00019B/871/P

To

Margaret

DESCENDING SOULS

Thanks for buying this book and the support. This is one of the original set published.

all the best,

John.